ASSESSMENT OF TUMOUR RESPONSE

DEVELOPMENTS IN ONCOLOGY 11

Previously published in this series:

1. F.J. Cleton and J.W.I.M. Simons, eds., Genetic Origins of Tumor Cells
   ISBN 90-247-2272-1
2. J. Aisner and P. Chang, eds., Cancer Treatment Research
   ISBN 90-247-2358-2
3. B.W. Ongerboer de Visser, D.A. Bosch and W.M.H. van Woerkom-Eykenboom, eds., Neuro-Oncology: Clinical and Experimental Aspects
   ISBN 90-247-2421-X
4. K. Hellmann, P. Hilgard and S. Eccles, eds., Metastasis: Clinical and Experimental Aspects
   ISBN 90-247-2424-4
5. H.F. Seigler, ed., Clinical Management of Melanoma
   ISBN 90-247-2584-4
6. P. Correa and W. Haenszel, eds., Epidemiology of Cancer of the Digestive Tract
   ISBN 90-247-2601-8
7. L.A. Liotta and I.R. Hart, eds., Tumor Invasion and Metastasis
   ISBN 90-247-2611-5
8. J. Bánóczy, ed., Oral Leukoplakia
   ISBN 90-247-2655-7
9. C. Tijssen, M. Halprin and L. Endtz, eds., Familial Brain Tumours
   ISBN 90-247-2691-3
10. F.M. Muggia, C.W. Young and S.K. Carter, eds., Anthracycline Antibiotics in Cancer
    ISBN 90-247-2711-1

Series ISBN: 90-247-2338-8

ASSESSMENT OF TUMOUR RESPONSE

edited by

B.W. HANCOCK, MD, DCH, MRCP,
Senior Lecturer in Medicine
Honorary Consultant Physician
Royal Hallamshire & Weston Park Hospitals,
Sheffield. U.K.

1982

MARTINUS NIJHOFF PUBLISHERS
THE HAGUE / BOSTON / LONDON

Distributors:

for the United States and Canada
Kluwer Boston, Inc.
190 Old Derby Street
Hingham, MA 02043
USA

for all other countries
Kluwer Academic Publishers Group
Distribution Center
P.O. Box 322
3300 AH Dordrecht
The Netherlands

Library of Congress Cataloging in Publication Data CIP

Main entry under title:

Assessment of tumour response.

(Developments in oncology ; 11)
Includes index.
1. Tumors--Treatment--Evaluation. I. Hancock, B. W.
II. Series: Developments in oncology; v. 11. [DNLM:
1. Neoplasm staging--Methods. 2. Neoplasms--Therapy.
W1 DE998N v.11 / QZ 241 A846]
RC270.8.A87 1982 616.99'407 82-18861
ISBN 90-247-2712-X

ISBN 90-247-2712-X (this volume)
ISBN 90-247-2338-8 (series)

PRINTED IN THE NETHERLANDS

Table of Contents

Preface

The assessment of tumour response after treatment is one of the most important challenges in Oncology and the picture is so often complicated by the effects of therapy itself. Clinical assessment is still by far the most important method of assessment at our disposal but there is increasing dependence on investigations of all types as indices of response. This dependence may be misplaced if inappropriate investigations are pursued and we have tried to emphasise in this book the importance of selectivity. Some indices of assessment (e.g. tumour markers, organ imaging) have a vital role to play; others (e.g. histopathology, genetics) are assuming greater importance as tumour behaviour becomes better understood. One subject, Immunology, is still in its infancy as regards tumour follow-up, but shows much promise so that a full account of tumour immunology and trends in immunotherapy has been included.

I am grateful to Dr. Brian Ross for his help with the chapter on Organ Imaging, to the Department of Medical Illustration for their ever-ready co-operation with illustrations and photographs and to Miss Shirley Francis for doing much of the typing.

B. W. HANCOCK

List of Contributors

HANCOCK, B. W., MD, DCH, MRCP, Senior Lecturer in Medicine, Honorary Consultant Physician, Royal Hallamshire & Weston Park Hospitals, Sheffield, U.K.

NEAL, F. E., KSG, MBChB, FRCR, DMRT, Consultant Radiotherapist & Oncologist, Weston Park Hospital, Sheffield, U.K.

POTTER, A.M., BSc, MMedSci, Principal Scientific Officer, Centre for Human Genetics, Sheffield, U.K.

POWELL, T., MB, BCh, FRCP, FRCR, DMRD, Consultant Radiologist, Royal Hallamshire & Weston Park Hospitals, Sheffield, U.K.

PRENTON, M. A., BA, MB, BChir, MSc, FRCPath, Consultant Chemical Pathologist, Royal Hospital, Chesterfield, U.K.

REES, R. C., BSc, PhD, Senior Lecturer in Virology, University of Sheffield Medical School, Sheffield, U.K.

RICHMOND, J., MD, FRCP, Professor of Medicine, Royal Hallamshire Hospital, Sheffield, U.K.

ROSS, C. M. D., MB, ChB, DCP, FRCPath, Senior Lecturer in Pathology, Honorary Consultant Pathologist, Royal Hallamshire and Weston Park Hospitals, Sheffield, U.K.

TOMLINSON, S., MD, MRCP, Reader in Medicine, Honorary Consultant Physician, Northern General Hospital, Sheffield, U.K.

UNDERWOOD, J. C. E., MD, MRCPath, Senior Lecturer in Pathology, Honorary Consultant Pathologist, Royal Hallamshire Hospital, Sheffield, U.K.

WARD, A. MILFORD, MA, MB, BChir, FRCPath, Senior Lecturer in Immunology, Director of Supraregional Protein Reference Unit, Royal Hallamshire Hospital, Sheffield, U.K.

1. Clinical Assessment

B. W. HANCOCK and F. E. NEAL

1. Clinical monitoring

Perhaps the most difficult aspect of clinical oncology is that of monitoring, which demands great experience as well as skill since the assessment is often complicated by side issues. The monitoring process, which must usually be continued for many years, is concerned basically with the assessment of the response of the tumour to a therapy. Several factors are helpful in making such an assessment (see Table 1) but often the judgment is made on empirical grounds. Certain rules have been accepted to enable comparable information to be produced and to enhance the management of patients. These rules are concerned with the objective assessment of response and are based on a standardised terminology regarding the degree of response. Although the use of such guidelines is to be encouraged, there are often limitations imposed by the clinical progress in a particular patient.

Table 1. Factors helpful in making an assessment of tumour response

1) The type and extent of the tumour at presentation
2) The presence of favourable or poor prognostic factors at presentation
3) The expected natural biological behaviour of such a tumour
4) The general well-being of the patient at presentation and during treatment
5) The rate and degree of response of the tumour to treatment
6) Objective measurement of clinical and investigative indices at regular intervals with accurate recording of data

Recommendations [1] on the standardisation of reporting results of cancer treatment have recently been published (under the auspices of the World Health Organisation). General principles have been suggested for the minimal requirements in assessing and recording baseline data (relating to patient, tumour and laboratory and radiological investigations), on reporting treatment, on grading acute and subacute toxicity, and on reporting response, recurrence, disease-free interval and other results of therapy. By using such principles the results from one centre should be comparable with those from any other in the world.

Success in the management of the patient with malignant disease is directed towards the complete and permanent eradication of the tumour

Hancock, B. W. (ed.), Assessment of Tumour Response.
 ISBN 90-247-2712-X.
Printed in The Netherlands.

mass with minimal damage to the patient, but it has to be accepted that this ideal will only be achieved in about 30% of patients in the present state of our knowledge. Much of the management, therefore, will be of a palliative nature and it is essential for the clinician to be able to define whether palliation has been achieved or not. Obviously there has to be some improvement in the patient's clinical state and an increase in the quality of life if a palliative improvement is to be claimed. In the attempt to eradicate a tumour, the clinician must be aware of the potential damage which accrues from the various treatment modalities and must remember that he is essentially concerned with the well-being of the patient rather than the treatment of a malignant mass. It is difficult to define end points of cancer therapy, and with the increasing use of combined modalities and more aggressive therapy, the incidence of side effects and complications is likely to rise. Unfortunately the long-term complications of some modern treatments have not yet been assessed because it is only as a particular treatment protocol becomes more successful in the way of long-term survival that late side effects are revealed. Thus a realistic compromise has to be established between achieving regression and the resulting damage. All treatment protocols in regular use carry a high incidence of adverse effects, and the clinician must be aware of all the possibilities following a particular treatment regime.

2. Methods of assessment of response

There is no substitute for clinical assessment and various monitoring procedures merely complement and enhance what the experienced clinician has discovered following his examination of the patient. He should be able to assess the patient's progress by merely listening to the history! The team approach to oncology is never more obvious than when applying the knowledge from multiple disciplines in the careful follow-up of patients. The roles of laboratory-based colleagues will be discussed in detail in later chapters but it is the clinician who sees the patient at each attendance and it is on his judgment that investigations are initiated.

3. Definition of response

There is still much variability in the accepted definitions of response but many authorities would agree with the following guidelines formulated by the UICC [2]; these were originally devised for use with breast carcinoma but can be applied with modifications to most other forms of cancer. The categories of response were defined simply as:

1) Complete response – disappearance of all evidence of disease as determined by two observations four or more weeks apart.
2) Partial response – 50% or more decrease in the size of some or all of measurable lesions and unequivocal improvement in other lesions, determined by two observations four or more weeks apart. No lesions should have progressed.
3) No response – 'static' disease, in which lesions either show less than 50% regression or minimal (less than 25%) progression and 'progressive' disease, in which most lesions progress despite treatment. Failure of therapy is when there is progression of existing lesions and appearance of new ones.

The term 'less-than-partial response' (where a reduction in size of 25–50% of tumour is recorded) has recently been introduced [3].

In association with these objective criteria for response, it is important to state the duration of complete response (complete objective remission) from the date that complete response is first recorded to the date of the first observation of progressive disease. This is in theory impossible to determine accurately because the start and end-point of the response are so difficult to define. The overall response period (complete or partial remission) is usually taken as the time from the start of treatment to the first finding of progressive disease and is therefore longer than, and must be distinguished from, the duration of complete response.

The minimum assessable response duration is generally taken as four weeks. This is, however, a woefully short time period, particularly in assessing partial or less-than-partial responses, when taking into account tumour growth kinetics; the growth and regression rates of human tumours are extremely variable, e.g. doubling times in different tumours vary from 10 days to 4 months [4].

Recurrence after treatment can be defined as the progression of residual disease or appearance of new disease in a previously treated area or the development of distant metastases. The assessment of recurrence again relies on multi-disciplinary assessment – clinical, histological and investigative criteria must be evaluated. Survival, overall and disease-free, from the time of commencing treatment until death, should be recorded in all cases.

One obvious ideal way to establish accurate criteria and data evaluation is by means of the randomised prospective multi-centre clinical trial [5] organised on the basis of a firm statistical grounding and posing few questions, all of which can be completely answered; ideally there should be a definite end-point. Failing this it is important for each centre to define firm criteria for tumour treatment and assessment of response, and to record data in such a way that these can be interpreted by other centres. The establishment of international anatomical classifications (e.g. TNM), pathological classifications and follow-up criteria (as discussed above) should provide a basis for such an ideal situation.

4. The clinician's role

There are clearly many pitfalls for the oncologist assessing tumour response [6] since this depends on the composition and growth kinetics of the tumour itself, on the actual measurement indices and, of course, on the quality of the clinical data.

The clinician who sees the patient at his initial presentation and supervises his initial management is obviously the ideal person to undertake follow-up. It is preferable, but not always possible, for the same clinician to see the patient at subsequent appointments, and if the original clinician is not available the patient should be seen by a member of the same clinical team.

The first essential is to establish an excellent rapport with the patient which will enhance management throughout the remainder of the clinical course of the patient's disease. This is ideally achieved at the initial consultation when the patient must be assured that the clinican has time to listen, assess, and communicate details of the proposed treatment. An accurate record of the history and examination is essential to provide baselines on which to graft future assessments particularly if the patient is to be seen by other clinicians. No matter how minor the malignant process, therefore, with the possible exception of small skin cancers, a complete clinical examination is mandatory, noting not only the extent of the primary lesion and the presence of metastases, but also the signs of coincidental disease which may be aggravated by subsequent treatment. The establishment of an ongoing rapport with the patient ensures that changes in general health and local problems will be willingly reported and an early consultation initiated if unexpected symptoms arise. Such is the fear of cancer in the community that many patients instinctively hide symptoms developing after treatment because they feel these are bound to indicate recurrence of disease. Constant reassurance is therefore essential.

If the patient is known to the clinician changes in general health will be obvious prior to full examination. Many patients complain of bizarre symptoms which at first sight appear irrelevant and may not relate to what is expected in a particular disease. These should not be ignored; the experienced oncologist will know that they often relate to subclinical spread which may not become overt for some time. Subtle changes in physical or psychological make-up can also be observed, which may be markers towards the extension of the malignant process. The oncologist will be guided by his knowledge of the biology and natural history of similar tumours and will be aware of the many possibilities relating to a particular symptom. The problem of mimicry is now a well-known hazard in cancer management and no symptom should be ignored! More concrete clinical criteria should be assessed. These include such things as change in appetite or weight, general health, relevant symptomatic enquiry, presence of systemic symptoms or signs (e.g. para-neoplastic disorders) and features such as pain relief and, most important, appreciation of changes in the tumour itself. The clinical assessment will involve measurement of visible and palpable lesions at regular intervals, the assessment of non-measurable but nevertheless evaluable lesions, and the institution of relevant investigations, taking into account the known probable pattern of spread of the tumour and the risk–benefit ratio of the investigation (i.e., do the results obtained from the test help in the management of the tumour without doing disproportionate harm to the patient?). Simple tests such as blood count, ESR and chest X-ray can be almost routine at follow-up; other more expensive, tedious and invasive or less accurate assessments must be judiciously and appropriately selected. Recurrence of tumour should be established on firm clinical or histological grounds. Changes in treatment with dates must be recorded meticulously; also important are the time and cause of death (determined whenever possible by autopsy) when this occurs.

Throughout follow-up the clinician may have difficulty in distinguishing the local and metastatic complications of cancer from the many side effects of treatment. It is also well recognised that many patients with cancer have specific and non-specific effects not attributable to the primary lesion or metastases. Some of these syndromes which may be dermatological [7], neurological [8] and endocrinological (see Chapter 5) are also difficult to differentiate from the effects of treatment. Since malignant disease is now accepted as the great mimic an accurate and wide-ranging knowledge of the tumour and its treatment is therefore vital, and any symptoms or sign should be assumed to be due to the tumour, or its treatment, unless proven otherwise (see Table 2).

A more difficult assessment is that of deciding when a mass is a recurrent tumour or not. In the situation where complete regression has been achieved the appearance at a later date of a mass, or in more difficult circumstances ill-defined induration, makes it essential for the clinician to know what the reappearance of 'abnormal tissue' implies. In most instances the only satisfactory way in which to resolve the problem is to adopt a watching policy – carefully assessing any changes at frequent intervals with measurement of size related to specifically designated points. The increase in size of such a mass is not in itself indicative of recurrent disease, and the experienced clinician will be aware that post-operative and especially post-radiation fibrosis, may often resemble recurrence. Eventually histological confirmation of the nature of the mass may be required but this often pre-

Table 2. Follow-up disorders that may be complications of the cancer or side effects of the treatment

Disorder	Complications of cancer	Side-effects of treatment
General malaise/anorexia/weight loss	Progressive tumour/poor nutrition/poor hydration	Short-term effect of RT & CT
Fever	Persistent tumour (particularly Hodgkins, renal, liver)	Infection (immunosuppression resulting from RT, CT)
Psychiatric	Stress { uncertain prognosis physical debility	Mastectomy, colostomy, chemophobia, alopecia
Nausea and vomiting	Feature of widespread tumour burden Mechanical effects of abdominal tumour	Short term effect of RT & CT
Bowel disturbance	Constipation in debilitated, immobile patient Mechanical effects of abdominal tumour	Diarrhoea (RT & CT) Constipation (e.g. vincristine) Adhesions (surgery ± radiotherapy)
Haematological	Marrow depression or infiltration, folate deficiency, haemolysis	Myelosuppression (CT, RT)
Dermatological	Infiltration, paraneoplastic conditions	Radiation and drug reactions Phlebitis/necrosis at iv site
Neurological	Metastases to brain and spinal cord Paraneoplastic syndromes	Neurotoxicity (vinca alkaloids, methotrexate, cis platinum) Myelitis (RT)
Renal	Obstruction from tumour Infiltration by tumour	Nephrotoxicity (e.g. cis platinum) Hyperuricaemia Radiation nephritis
Hepatic	Infiltration by tumour Portal obstruction by tumour nodes	Hepatotoxicity (e.g. methotrexate) Hepatitis
Respiratory	Lung metastases. Pleural effusion	Lung fibrosis (RT, bleomycin) Opportunistic infection
Cardiac	Cardiac infiltration. Pericardial effusion	Cardiomyopathy (doxorubicin, daunorubicin) Constrictive pericarditis (RT)
Electrolytic	1) Consequence of renal/liver infiltration 2) Nutritional debility/dehydration 3) Ectopic hormone effects ((ACTH, ADH, Ca^{++})	Dehydration (RT, CT, surgery)

RT: radiotherapy; CT: chemotherapy.

sents a hazard because there is a danger of causing further damage by an over-enthusiastic approach to biopsy. Although the establishment of a definite diagnosis of a mass may be of interest, the desire for definite fact should be tempered with the need to know what can be done about a recurrence if it is confirmed.

4.1. Specific symptoms

There are certain specific symptoms which may be invaluable in assessment.

4.1.1. Tiredness is inevitable following all forms of therapy but this should be a temporary phenomenon and should disappear once a tumour has been controlled. Reappearance of tiredness, especially in the absence of other signs of activity, should be regarded as an important symptom and may be the first sign of impending recurrence. However, it is important to differentiate between the general lethargy of disease and the depression which some patients experience at various times in the course of their illness. The latter is a reflection of their underlying anxiety resulting from their awareness of the diagnosis and may occur even when they are free of disease.

4.1.2. Anorexia is an important symptom which is produced by disease or by treatment. As with tiredness, it should be transient and its recurrence is usually an indication that the malignant process is again active. Failure to gain weight may result from a number of features [9] – anorexia, depression, mechanical interference with feeding (which may occasionally complicate treatment), malabsorption, protein loss, hepatic insufficiency, ectopic hormone syndromes associated with weight loss and cancer cachexia. Nutritional assessment and maintenance with correction of dehydration and electrolyte abnormalities is therefore a vital part of follow-up and tumour reassessment.

4.1.3. Pain is often used as an empirical marker of tumour recurrence and in many instances it is an important warning sign. Pain may occur at the primary site due to infiltration of surrounding tissues but is also produced by pressure on nerve roots or by the occurrence of metastases in a distant site. Bone pain is a common complaint and usually results from the presence of metastases. However, the pain may be due to coincidental disease or complication of treatment and is not uncommonly associated with post-operative or post-radiation fibrosis, and bone pain may occasionally occur as a result of radiation changes within bone. Differentiation between recurrence and complication is often difficult and multiple investigations may be required.

4.1.4. Nausea and vomiting complicate most cancer treatments but should be transient phenomena. Recurrence of these symptoms in an apparently healthy patient, however, should give rise to concern. These symptoms are often non-specifically indicative of general ill health but may be caused by more specific syndromes, e.g. hypercalcaemia, which is a common termination of some cancers. There is also the vomiting associated with raised intracranial pressure in cerebral metastases. As a late phenomenon of treatment, these symptoms are seen usually in conjunction with recurrent malignant disease involving the gastrointestinal tract or where treatment has produced damage.

4.1.5. Dyspnoea may indicate active disease or may be a complication of treatment. It is a common problem after treatment of patients with bronchial carcinoma and usually indicates active disease; it may however be a symptom of the persistent anaemia which often complicates malignant disease or as a sequel of radiation therapy to the chest or following the use of certain cytotoxic agents. The assessment of the importance of this symptom in a particular patient is very difficult, not easily resolved by investigation, and often it is necessary to rely on the subsequent clinical course to provide the answer.

4.1.6. Haemorrhage may be a prominent symptom in patients attending for follow-up. Neoplastic processes usually only produce bleeding if there has been invasion of a blood vessel or if a large ulcerated area is present, either externally or within a viscus, from which surface oozing takes place. To complicate the problem, bleeding is also a sequela of radiation therapy – arising from telangiectatic vessels and with certain cytotoxic agents, e.g. cyclophosphamide, which cause damage to the epithelium of the urinary tract. Diagnosis is usually simple and can be deduced from a careful consideration of the history but occasionally investigations are required.

4.1.7. Fever is undoubtedly a feature of many tumours [10] (particularly lymphomas, leukaemias and kidney, liver and Ewing's tumours). It is probably derived from a tumour product acting directly on the central nervous system or inducing production of an endogenous pyrogen from reticulo-endothelial cells [11]. Once treatment has started, however, fever is more likely to be due to infection and the immunosuppressive and myelosuppressive effects of cancer therapy are well recognised. A careful search for opportunistic infection (bacterial, viral, fungal or protozoal) is therefore vital;

energetic and early treatment of septicaemia may be life-saving. The old idea of tumour necrosis causing fever, particularly following therapy, has little to support it unless there is localised infection (e.g. abscess formation) within the tumour itself.

4.1.8. Psychological problems are not uncommon with certain types of cancer [12] – affective disorders, organic brain syndromes, childhood behaviour problems and sexual problems are all seen. These disorders are in part due to the stress of the cancer (physical debility, uncertainty of prognosis), to the effects of treatment (e.g. mastectomy and alopecia in patients with breast tumours, colostomy after bowel surgery, chemophobia in patients attending for regular 'upsetting' chemotherapy regimes) and to the anxieties of follow-up (the worry about the success or failure of the treatment). The quality of life in patients, and their relatives, should be monitored [12] and prompt recognition and referral of psychiatric problems with appropriate assessment and treatment is obviously important.

4.2.. Clinical examination

Although the changes in symptomatology may indicate active disease the most important part of clinical assessment is provided by a detailed examination of the patient with careful reference to earlier records. Clinical examination is directed towards the primary lesion and the sites of possible metastases.

4.2.1. Ulceration. Local ulceration at the site of the original tumour is not necessarily indicative of recurrent disease. Although always a cause for concern it must be interpreted carefully. Though not common, radiation changes induced at the time of treatment will jeopardise blood supply and subsequent ulceration may indicate necrosis rather than recurrence. Similarly, the fibrosis which can occur following treatment may result in ill-defined induration which can mimic disease. Whilst the difference is usually obvious, there are occasions when there is difficulty in establishing the correct diagnosis and it is necessary to resort to histological examination.

4.2.2. Changes in colouration. Extending tumour may invade the skin and by slow infiltration cause changes which produce a characteristic colouration. Usually such changes are accompanied by the presence of a mass and the underlying pathology is not in doubt. Radiation treatment may also produce changes which, together with underlying fibrosis, may lead to confusion. Some progressive tumours may produce generalised changes in pigmentation which can occasionally be mimicked by the effects of cytotoxic, hormonal or radiation therapy. Care is required therefore in the assessment of such changes and the subsequent clinical course is usually sufficient to resolve the problem.

4.2.3. Infection. Local or systemic infection may cause problems. Obviously large ulcerated areas may become infected but infection is a common accompaniment of active tumour, and occasionally of treatment, in closed cavities especially around the head and neck and in pelvic disease. Infection in bone can give rise to troublesome symptoms and may be seen following irradiation especially if further trauma to the bone occurs (e.g. dental extraction).

5. The role of surgery

Staging surgery is now an accepted essential part of the initial assessment of patients with cancer and is likely to become more important as our knowledge of specific malignancies extends. 'Second look' surgery, perhaps even as a repeated procedure, will be used increasingly in the monitoring of patients, e.g. with lymphoma and certain ovarian, testicular and gastro-intestinal tumours, complementing clinical surveillance to determine whether disease has been eradicated or if further therapy is required.

6. Surveillance

It is obvious that the after care of patients with cancer is of the greatest importance and must be performed carefully and accurately if optimum management is to be achieved. The frequency of follow-up is a vital matter and should be determined according to the curability of the particular type of tumour (Table 3). Thus where there is real probability of cure and further treatment is possible if recurrence or metastases occur, frequent follow-up is indicated in the early stages after treatment, the intervals between examinations lengthening with the passage of time. Where cure is less probable and a palliative type of management has been employed, it is preferable to extend the intervals between follow-up appointments as rapidly as possible in order to spare the patient the unnecessary journey for a pointless consultation. There is little point in looking for activity unless there is a further useful method of treatment available. If further problems develop in such patients it is a simple matter for the general medical practitioner to return them to the specialist clinic before the appointed day, or for the patient to initiate a consultation.

Table 3. Follow-up according to tumour type

Potentially curable cancers	Children's tumours Lymphoma Testicular tumours Acute leukaemia S.C.C. of ear, nose & throat Thyroid tumours Uterine tumours Carcinoma of skin	Frequent follow-up in the period immediately after treatment, e.g. monthly. Gradually extending time if no evidence of active disease.
Intermediate. Tumours with long natural history which may or may not be curable	Ovarian cancer Renal tumours Carcinoma of breast Some melanomas Some sarcomas	Do not require frequent follow-up because of slow tumour growth. See reasonably frequently, e.g. two monthly initially. Can be extended if no evidence of activity.
Incurable cancers	Bronchus Bowel Brain	Usually rapidly fatal. Follow-up mainly for psychological reasons at long intervals.

Monitoring of all patients suffering from malignant disease should continue until there is no possibility of recurrence or until death from whatever cause. In most instances this means attendance at follow-up clinics for the rest of their life. The value of such an arrangement is disputed and should be carefully considered by individual clinicians before a definite commitment is made (Table 4). Eventually follow-up appointments are made for yearly intervals which is probably the only realistic long-term appointment, but many clinical changes may occur during a twelve-month period without the patient returning to his original clinician, so that vital information and the possibility of treatment is lost. On the other hand it would be quite impossible to see all patients at frequent intervals throughout the follow-up period and a suitable compromise must be made. If the patient remains in the follow-up clinic valuable statistic information will be obtained. Another important reason for continuing follow-up is to gain knowledge of the complications of treatment and to be able to initiate therapy in the presence of a second primary tumour.

The attendance of the patient at the specialised clinic can sometimes be a traumatic experience, causing psychological problems. Although there is a need for the clinical oncologist to see the patient in order to maintain continuity of management, other clinicians should be involved in the follow-up procedure. Ideally the patient should be seen regularly by his own family practitioner and returned to the clinic for relatively infrequent appointments. As well as saving the patient time and travelling problems, such a system would enhance patient care, relieving the oncologist from seeing fit

Table 4. Value of monitoring after therapy

For	Against
Psychologically helpful, e.g. patients gain confidence from knowing that they are having medical supervision	Psychologically harmful, e.g. may cause phobias
Assume that finding early disease will give better response to further treatment	Not always effective – may miss signs and ignore symptoms
Patients are more likely to return to a definite appointment than report back if symptoms develop	Changes may occur between appointments and patients may not report back
May detect pre-symptomatic disease	Inconvenient for the patient
Better patient care	Time consuming
Valuable statistics obtained by following up all patients	May have no effective treatment if active disease is discovered
	Increasing workload. Will follow up 'cured' patients

patients and allowing those for whom further advice is required to be assessed appropriately. It would also provide a psychological boost to the patient as well as optimum care. In this ideal situation the main load of monitoring would therefore fall on the general practitioner who would, of course, require accurate records of the patient's original assessment and therapy and would have to be aware of the various problems of the surveillance of patients with malignant disease.

References

1. Miller AB, Hoogstraten B, Staquet M, Winkler A: Reporting results of cancer treatment. Cancer 47:207–214, 1981.
2. Haywood JL, Carbone PP, Heuson JC, Kumaoka S, Segaloff A, Rubens RD: Assessment of response to therapy in advanced breast cancer. Cancer 39:1289–1294, 1977.
3. Gutterman JU, Blumenschein GR, Alexanian R, et al.: Leukocyte interferon induced tumour regression in human metastatic breast cancer, multiple myeloma and malignant lymphoma. Ann Intern Med 93:399–406, 1980.
4. Breur K: Growth rate and radiosensitivity of human tumours I. Growth rate of human tumours. Eur J Cancer 2:157–171, 1966.
5. Peto R: Monitoring patients in clinical trials, pp 377–381. In: Cancer: assessment and monitoring, Symmington T, Williams AE, McVie JG (eds). Edinburgh: Churchill Livingstone, 1980.
6. Watson JV: What does 'response' in cancer chemotherapy really mean? Br Med J 283:34–37, 1981.
7. Staughton RCD: Cutaneous manifestations of malignancy. Br J Hosp Med 20:38–47, 1978.
8. Croft P: Neuromuscular syndromes associated with malignant disease. Br J Hosp Med 17:356–362, 1977.

9. Editorial. Nutrition and the patient with cancer. Br Med J 2:846–847, 1978.
10. Editorial. Fever in malignant disease. Br Med J 1:591–592, 1974.
11. Young CW: Studies on fever in malignant disease, pp 235–241. In: Fever, Lipton JM (ed). New York: Raven Press, 1980.
12. Maguire P: Psychiatric aspects of malignant disease. SK and F Publications 4(2):1–12, 1981.

2. Organ Imaging

T. POWELL

1. Introduction

Until the end of the 19th century, the only effective means of tumour management was surgical excision. The decision for or against surgery was made on the clinical evidence as there could be no recourse to organ imaging. The discovery of X-rays by Röentgen in 1895 allowed both a new means of diagnosis, and a new method of treatment. Effective therapeutic use of radiation cannot, however, be made without some prior knowledge of the size, shape, position and nature of the lesion to be treated. Thus the science of organ and tumour imaging developed in part to service the need for effective radiotherapy. The subsequent development of new modalities of imaging including radio-isotope imaging, diagnostic ultrasound, and computed tomography greatly enhance the means by which a tumour may be defined. Further improvements may lie in the future with the development of nuclear magnetic resonance imaging (NMR) and positron emission tomography (PET). In addition, it is apparent that the information thus obtained, while allowing the clinician to plan treatment with greater accuracy, also allows for the assessment and follow up of the response to the treatment employed. Thus organ imaging is an important part of tumour management at the present time; the response to treatment, whether by radiation or chemotherapy, may be monitored by such means as are most appropriate to the tumour and organ in question. Also, there is a need to monitor the progress of secondary changes in affected organs and systems, including the urinary tract, liver, and lungs.

The importance of different imaging modalities is in a state of re-appraisal at the present time, because of the progressive introduction of facilities for computed tomography (CT) and the widespread availability of facilities for ultrasound and radio-isotope examination. While such techniques as conventional tomography and lymphography have been invaluable in the past, it has been long appreciated that there are inherent limitations which are to a considerable degree overcome by the newer techniques. In addition, it is often the case that the newer methods are not only more effective but less time-consuming and more pleasant for the patient than those they

Hancock, B. W. (ed.), Assessment of Tumour Response.
ISBN 90-247-2712-X.
Printed in The Netherlands.

replace. Unfortunately the cost of the apparatus necessary to perform these examinations is considerably greater than the cost of the devices they replace. The imaging service accounts for a substantial proportion of the cost of running an oncological unit.

The most appropriate modalities of imaging are selected according to the organ involved and the nature of the neoplastic process. Ideally all should offer a possibility of measuring tumour volume, but only in selected areas is this possible and the various compromises adopted are described below. Where, however, a mass of tumour is clearly demarcated, whether in a lymph node or in the lung, it may be used as a general indicator of the response to a treatment regime.

2. Lung tumours

Many lung tumours, both primary and secondary, are diagnosed by radiological methods. The evidence of such tumours may consist of a mass, atelectasis either partial or complete, or evidence of infection distal to an obstructive lesion in a bronchus. Peripheral tumour masses, and those not causing complete bronchial obstruction may be clearly imaged (Fig. 1a), and their response to treatment may be easily observed (Fig. 1b). However, these conditions apply to only a minority of patients with primary bronchial carcinoma. The difficulty arises in the separation of solid tissue in the thorax due to tumour from that due to secondary pulmonary collapse and infection lying in close anatomical relationship to the tumour. Conventional chest radiography, even when supplemented by tomography in the coronal, sagittal and transverse planes is limited in its ability to image the margins of many cases of bronchial carcinoma (Fig. 2). It is sometimes possible to resolve these small differences in radiographic tissue density by the use of computed tomography, but it remains true that the accurate delineation of a bronchial carcinoma cannot be achieved in many cases. From this it is clear that similar difficulties will apply in the assessment of the response of a bronchial neoplasm to treatment, the regression or otherwise of a tumour mass being to some extent masked by unresolved collapse, infection, radiation pneumonitis, and ultimately radiation fibrosis (Fig. 3). Tumour imaging agents such as gallium 67 have failed in general to establish a place in the assessment of primary bronchial carcinoma.

Pulmonary metastases present a different radiological problem in that they generally occur in the periphery of the lung. When they occur centrally in lymph nodes in the hila they do not for the most part cause bronchial obstruction, and their outline is therefore not masked by adjacent pulmon-

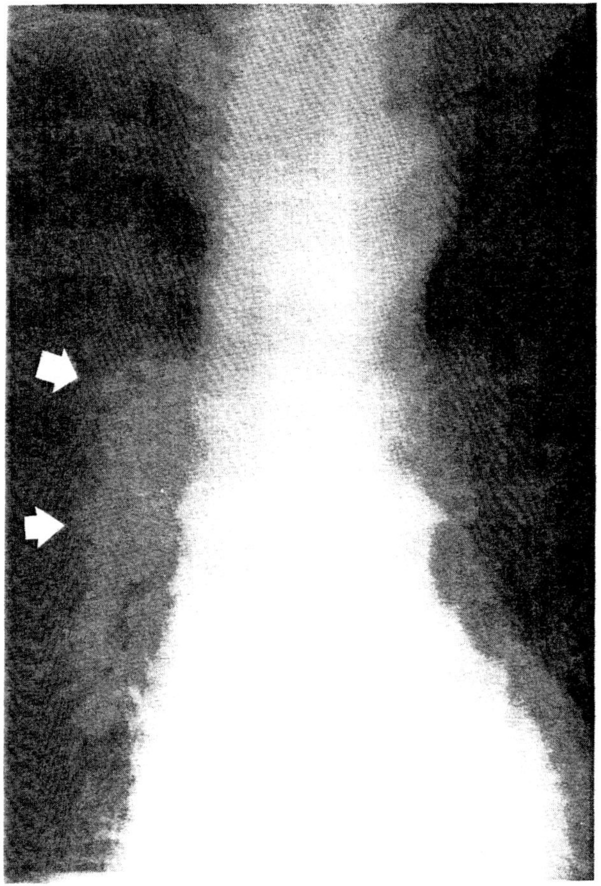

Figure 1a. Carcinoma of bronchus: tumour in R. hilum.

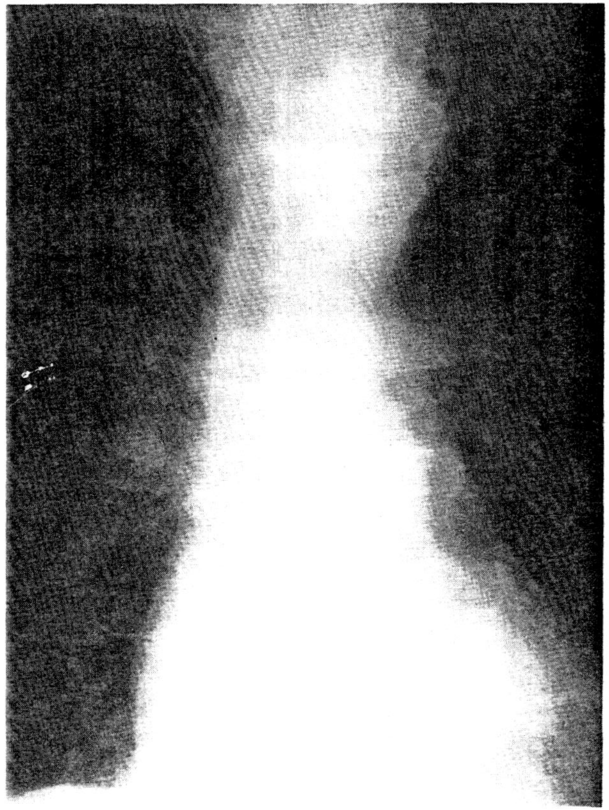

Figure 1b. Disappearance of tumour six weeks after radiotherapy.

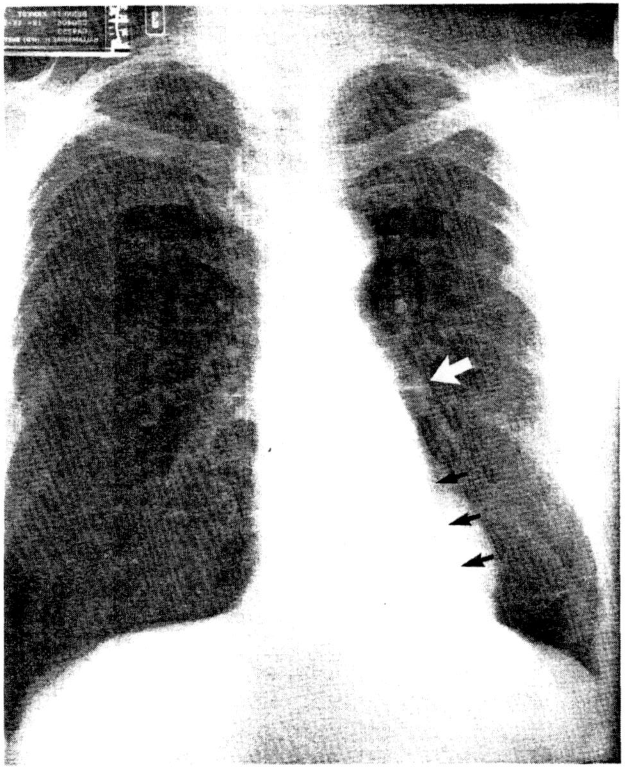

Figure 2. Collapse L. lower lobe due to hilar neoplasm. Only the lateral margin of tumour can be defined as the remainder is in contact with the mediastinum and with collapsed lung.

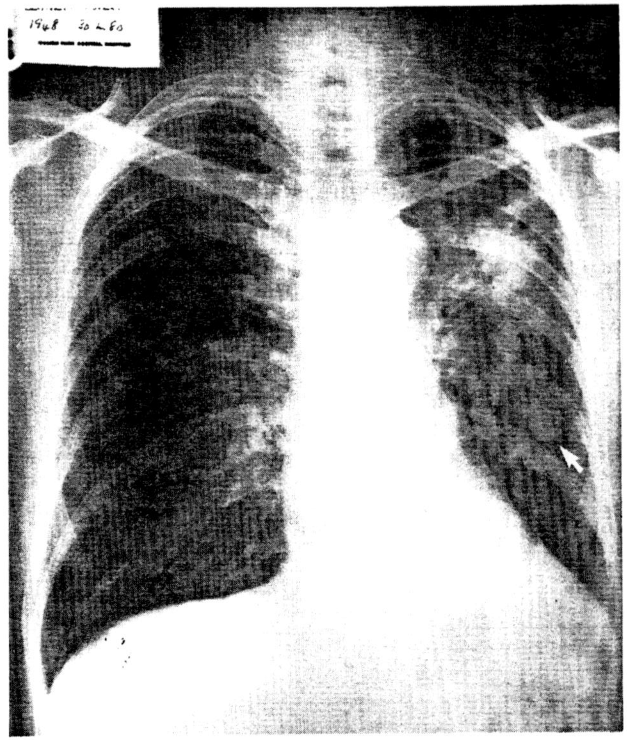

Figure 3. Same patient as in Fig. 2, four months after radiotherapy. Fibrosis, infection, and residual collapse tend to obscure residual or recurrent tumour. Nevertheless, a metastasis is visible (↖)

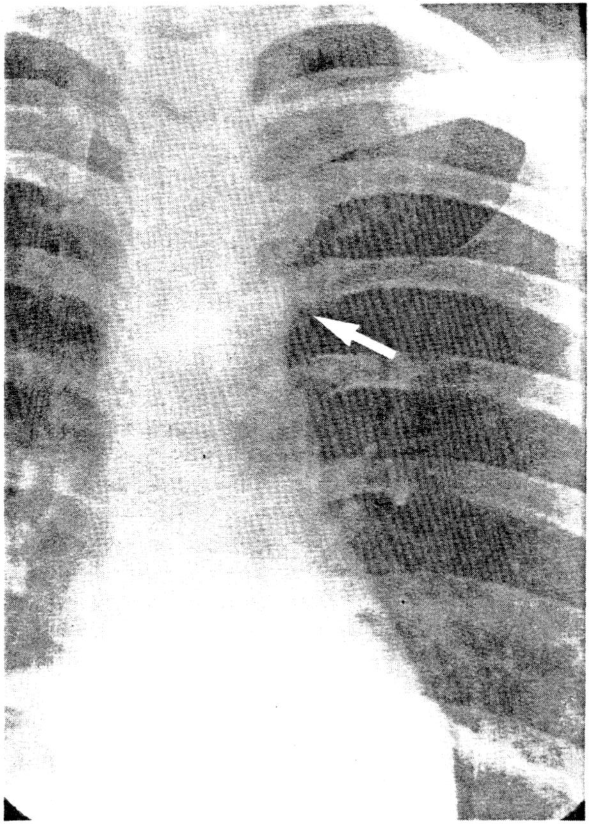

Figure 4a. Chorionepithelioma. Vague opacity contiguous with aortic knuckle.

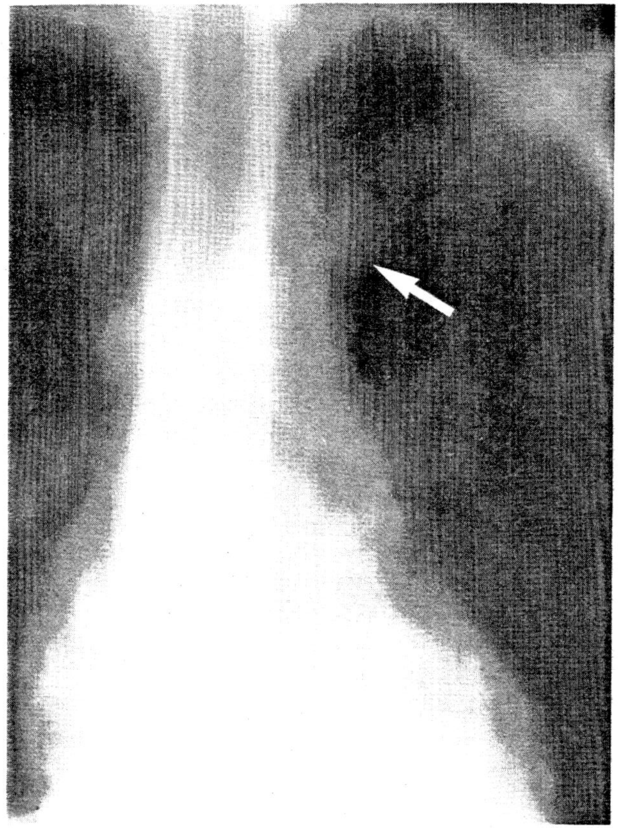

Figure 4b. Tomography clearly shows solitary tumour deposit.

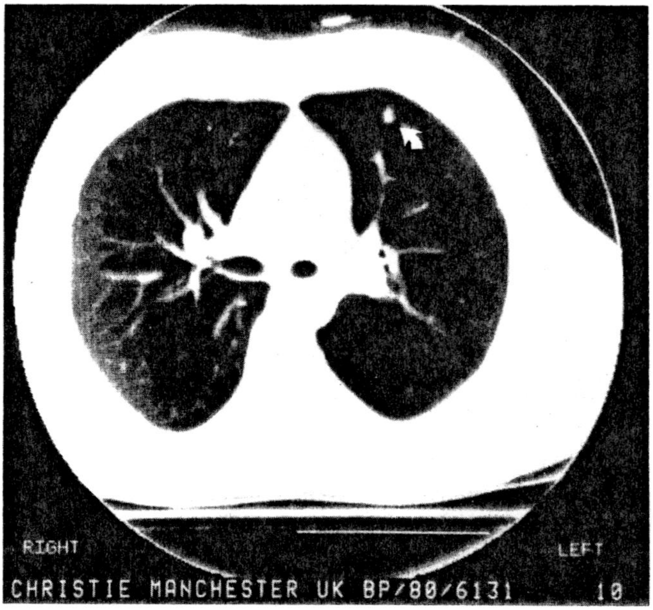

Figure 5. CT scan showing small metastases from a testicular teratoma (courtesy of Dr. B.J. Eddlestone, Christie Hospital, Manchester).

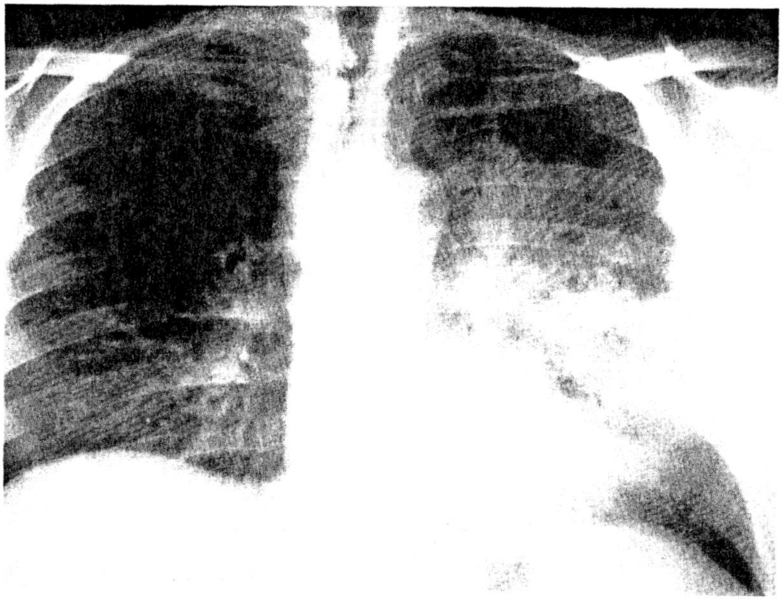

Figure 6a. Hodgkin's disease: infiltrative lesion L. lung.

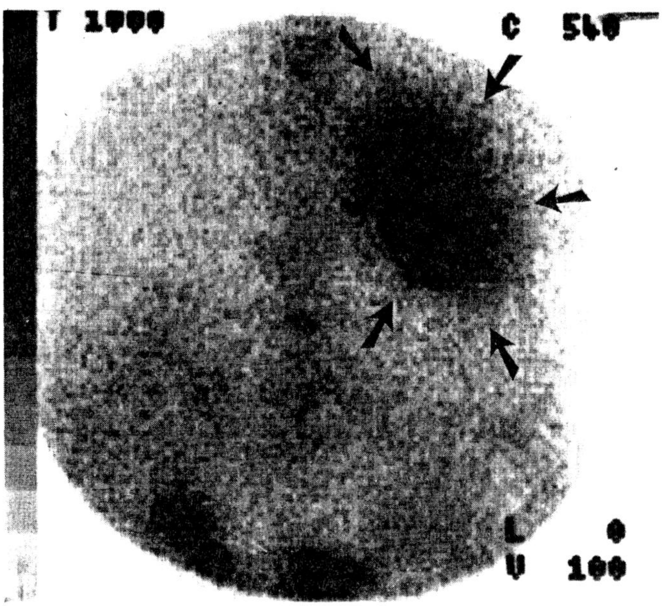

Figure 6b. Uptake of Gallium 67 in lesion in L. lung.

ary abnormalities. Many metastases appear on conventional radiographs, but the detection rate may be enhanced by the use of whole lung tomography (Figs. 4a, b). An even higher percentage of such metastases may be revealed by computed tomography (Fig. 5). In one series almost 30% of metastases in patients with testicular teratoma not visualised by whole lung tomography were demonstrated by CT [1]. In the same series the increased effectiveness of CT in the demonstration of mediastinal metastases was also described. CT is essential in those infrequent cases where excision of a presumed solitary pulmonary metastasis is contemplated following apparently successful eradication of a primary tumour. Such procedures are sometimes carried out in patients with a primary bone neoplasm or with a testicular teratoma.

The radio-isotope imaging of tumours in the lungs is more limited in its scope. Thyroid tumours not infrequently metastasise to the lung and, if they retain hormonal activity, may be imaged by thyroid seeking agents such as iodine 131 (see section 7).

Tumour tissues, particularly the lymphomata, have a particular affinity for gallium 67 which may be used in the diagnosis of lung infiltrates (Figs. 6a, b). Parenchymal involvement of the lung may be detected before it is visible on the radiographs [2]. Unfortunately the technique does not distinguish between inflammatory and neoplastic lung infiltrates.

Pleural and extra-pleural tumours both primary and secondary may be imaged on standard or oblique radiographs, and CT scanning is also of considerable value. Deposits may become obscured when there is associated pleural fluid, a frequent complication, and removal of the fluid may reveal otherwise obscured lesions. Introduction of air into the pleural cavity whether intentional or inadvertent is sometimes helpful in demonstrating pleural deposits.

3. Mediastinum

Tumours in the mediastinum, both primary and secondary, may be seen on plain radiographs, and it may in this site be easy to observe the effect of treatment (Figs. 7a, b). Tomography is of value for the hilar and subcarinal regions and also for the superior mediastinum (Figs. 8a, b). CT scanning is also effective in the detection of enlarged mediastinal and retrosternal lymph nodes, and in addition may show enlargement of the thymus [3]. There may be difficulty in distinguishing between the normal vascular structures of the mediastinum and enlarged lymph nodes, and in these cases contrast enhanced CT scans are of value.

Scanning of the mediastinum using gallium 67 may be of value in the lymphomas, demonstrating mediastinal disease in up to 28% of cases with negative radiographs [2]. The false negative rate appears to be very small. Hodgkin's and non-Hodgkin's lymphomas are equally well demonstrated. Confirmation of the significance of an apparently abnormal area of uptake may be obtained by recording the disappearance of the abnormality following appropriate treatment (Figs. 9a, b, c). Thyroid tumour metastases in the mediastinum may be imaged using thyroid seeking agents such as iodine 131 (see section 7).

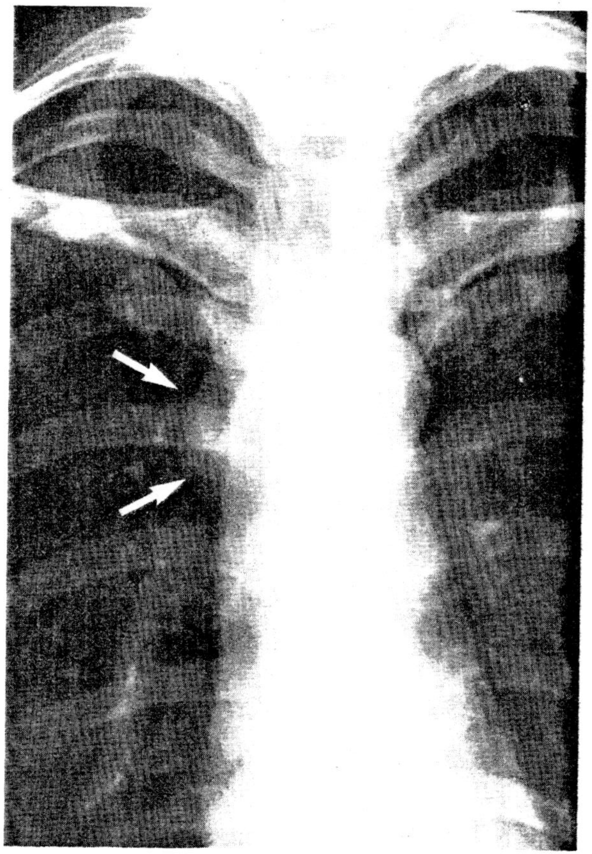

Figure 7a. Teratoma testis: metastasis in a right paratracheal lymph node.

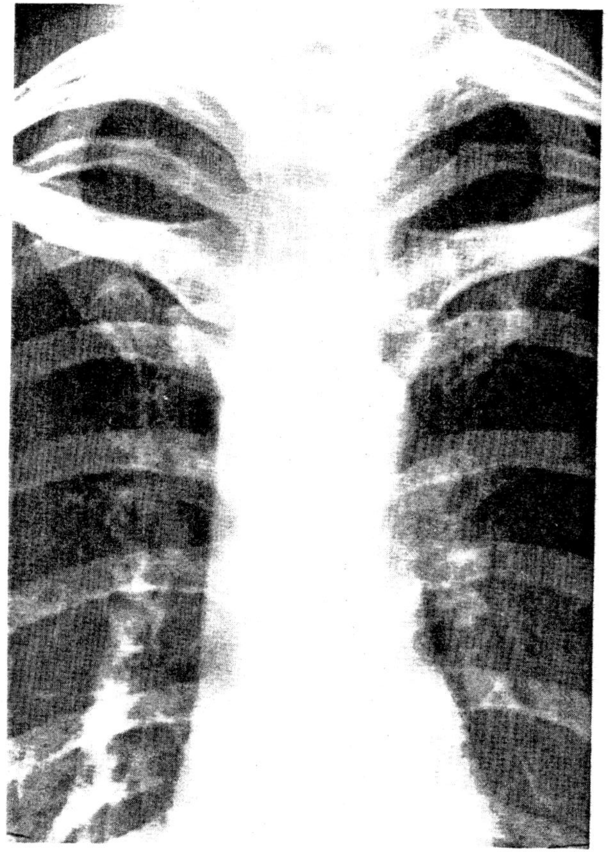

Figure 7b. Disappearance of mass four weeks after chemotherapy.

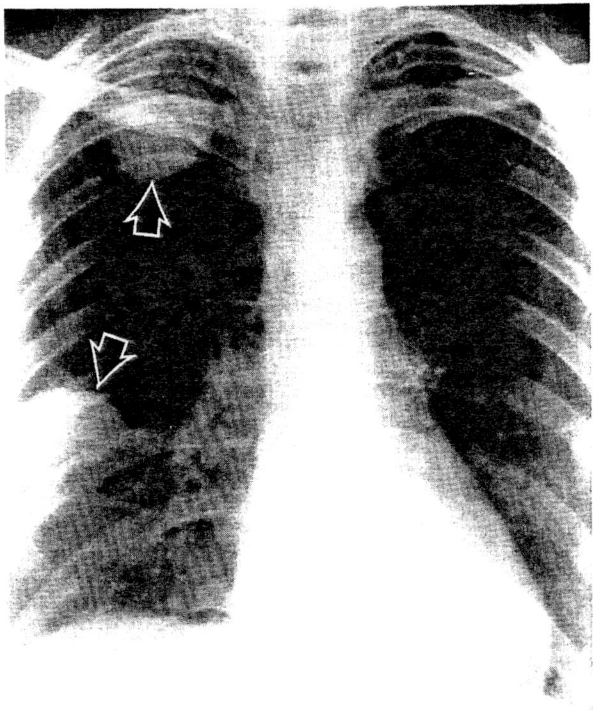

Figure 8a. Carcinoma of cervix: obvious lung metastases, but no mediastinal deposits seen.

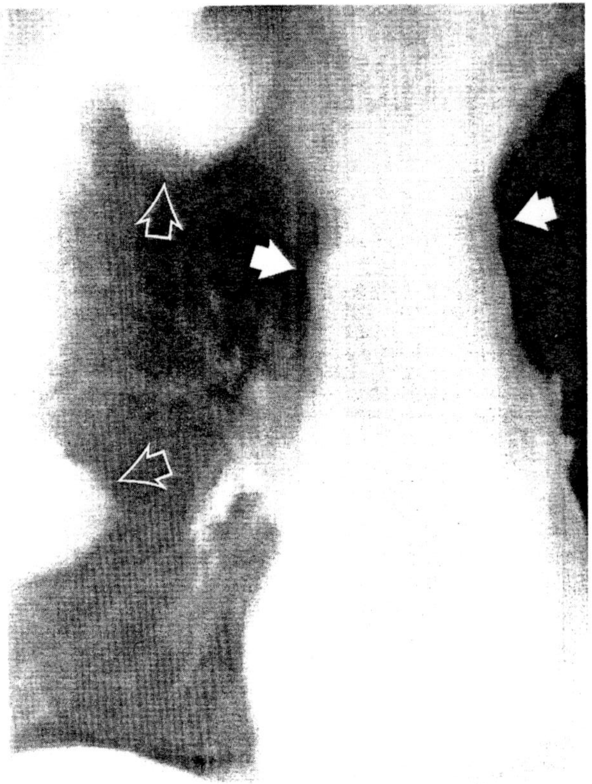

Figure 8b. Tomography additionally showing mediastinal lymph node metastases.

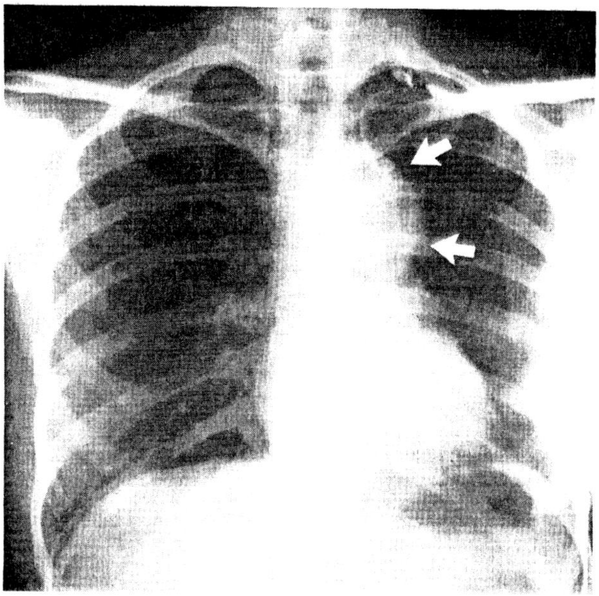

Figure 9a. Hodgkin's disease: mediastinal mass.

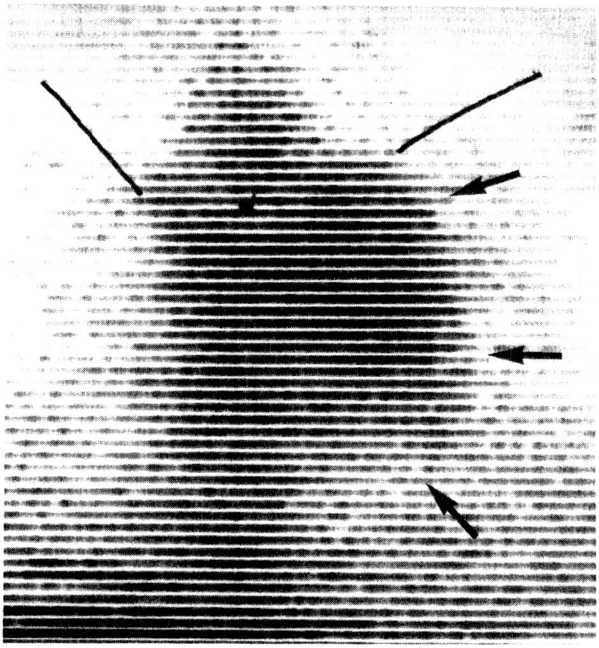

Figure 9b. Gallium 67 scan showing uptake in mass.

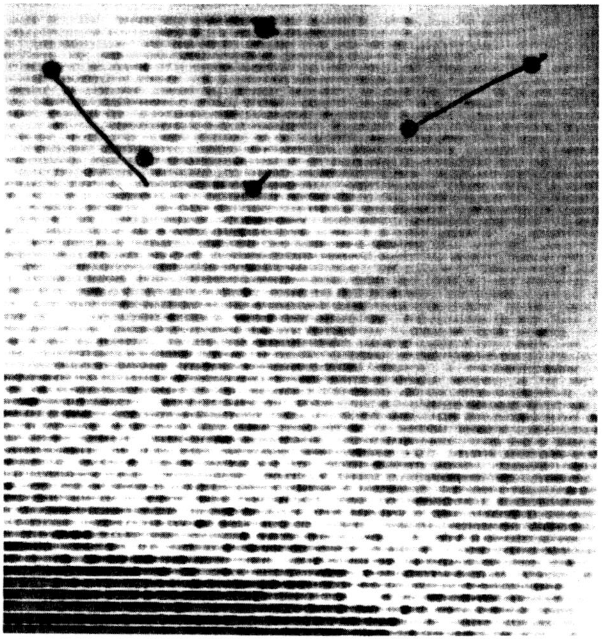

Figure 9c. Disappearance of area of Gallium 67 uptake six weeks after chemotherapy.

4. Abdominal lymph nodes

The assessment of the presence of metastatic malignant tumours and of lymphomatous infiltration in the abdominal lymph node chains is often a vital part of tumour staging and assessment of response. Despite the introduction of more modern techniques, lymphography is still widely practised. The contrast medium employed is an iodized oil of low viscosity injected into lymphatics on the dorsum of the feet by a technique originally developed by Kinmonth [4]. Limitations of the technique include failure to opacify the obturator and internal iliac lymph nodes, the lymph nodes in the mesentery and around the coeliac axis, those lying in the hila of the liver, spleen and kidneys, and those lying above the second lumbar vertebra including the retro-crural lymph nodes. Further difficulties arise because of concurrent chronic inflammatory changes, particularly in the inguinal and lower external iliac lymph nodes. Reactive changes may occur due to infection or following surgery, and may be difficult to distinguish from malignant infiltration. Extensive lymph node abnormalities may also be found in the collagenoses and in sarcoidosis. Despite these numerous difficulties lymphography has been widely practised for the staging and management of the lymphomas [5, 6, 7], tumours of the testis [8, 9], of the cervix and corpus uteri [10, 11] and of the bladder [12, 13, 14]. There has been a more limited acceptance of the value of lymphography in the management of tumours of the vulva and vagina, ovary, prostate and kidney, and in melanoma. The value of lymphography stems not only from its ability to demonstrate the presence of tumour within a lymph node, but because of its value in follow-up. The injected contrast medium will remain within a lymph node in assessable quantities for a year or even longer, enabling assessment of the response to treatment and also the detection of any subsequent recurrence [15]. Even traces of contrast medium may be sufficient for an assessment.

Normal lymph nodes appear as sharply demarcated elliptical structures having a finely granular pattern. Pathological lymph nodes are usually enlarged becoming reticular in appearance in the lymphomas (Fig. 10). There may be a small number of patients in whom nodes of normal size containing lymphoma deposits may be recognised as structurally abnormal on lymphography [5]. In metastatic tumours abnormal lymph nodes also tend to be enlarged but contain more discrete filling defects (Fig. 11). The lower external iliac and inguinal lymph nodes must be assessed with caution because of the frequent occurrence of chronic inflammatory changes producing filling defects due to fibro-fatty replacement. Urography is frequently carried out as an adjunct to lymphography, both for the assessment of the urinary tract (see below) and because the associated occurrence of ureteric displacement may aid in the assessment of the lymphogram (Fig. 12). This is particularly the case where there is uncertainty as to whether a gap in a lymph node chain is the result of an anatomical variant or due to a tumour replaced node. In the case of the latter there may be associated ureteric displacement. Re-examination at intervals may reveal the development of disease in lymph nodes originally thought to be normal (Figs. 13a, b) or may show regression of tumour deposits or infiltrates in lymph nodes seen to be diseased on the original radiographs (Figs. 14a, b). It should be noted that the response of a tumour to treatment is not necessarily accompanied by return of the lymph nodes to normal since the tumour deposits may become fibrotic. It is, therefore, inevitable that there are residual lymph node abnormalities, though lymph node enlargement usually disappears. It is also necessary to take into account the change in appearance due to clearance of contrast medium when assessing any abnormalities of internal structure of lymph nodes in the months following lymphography. The initial fairly

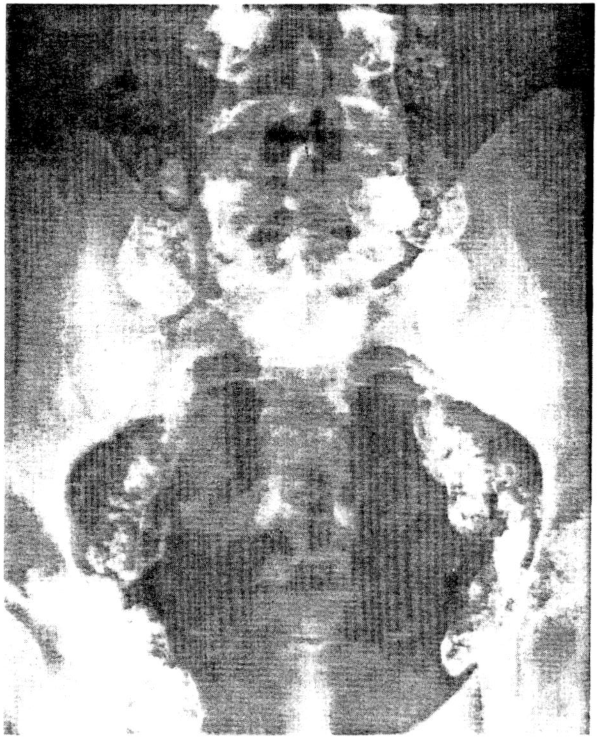

Figure 10. Enlarged lymph nodes showing reticular, or foamy structure: Hodgkin's disease.

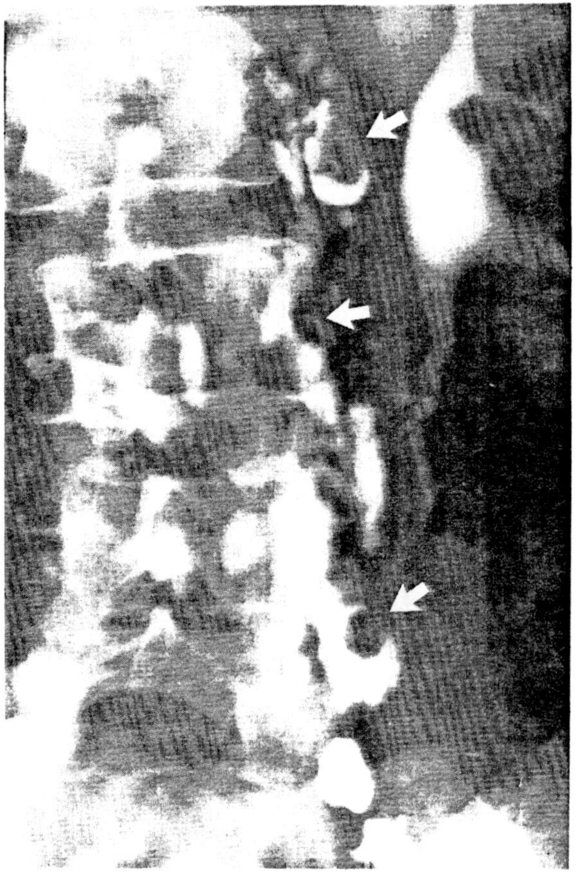

Figure 11. Lymph nodes containing discrete deposits: carcinoma of corpus uteri.

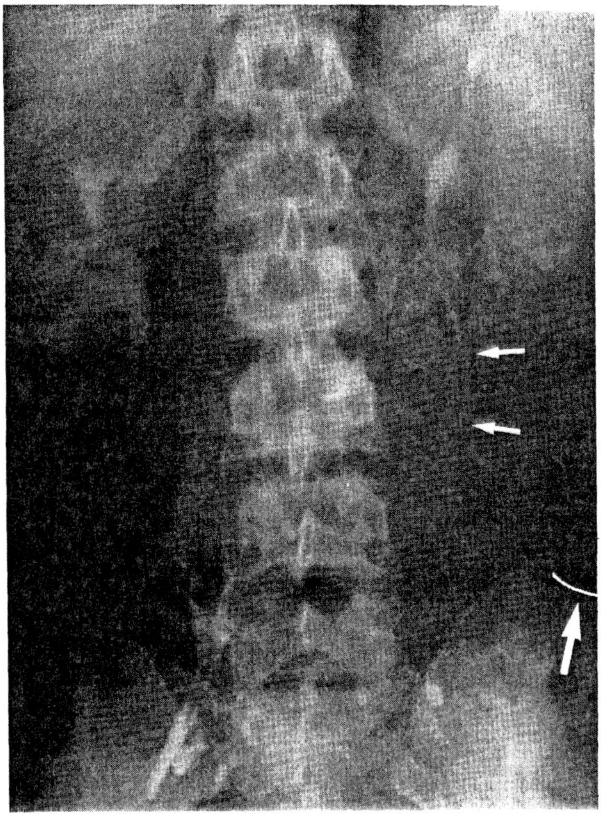

Figure 12. Hodgkin's disease: lymphogram shows marked lymph node enlargement. Note ureteric displacement (←). See also splenomegaly (↗).

homogenous appearance gives way to a more open texture as the contrast medium disappears. Magnification techniques [16] may occasionally be helpful in obtaining a more definitive diagnosis. In the lymph node areas opacified at lymphography, the accuracy rate in the lymphomas exceeds 90% [5, 6, 7].

It is apparent, however, from many lymphoma studies that conventional staging procedures including lymphography, seriously under-estimate the occurrence and extent of lymph node disease in the abdomen. It is also apparent that in some cases there may be an over-estimate, particularly in those patients with more advanced lymphomas. It is for these reasons that a diagnostic staging laparotomy has been widely adopted [17, 18, 19], this also enabling a more accurate determination to be made of possible involvement of the liver and spleen.

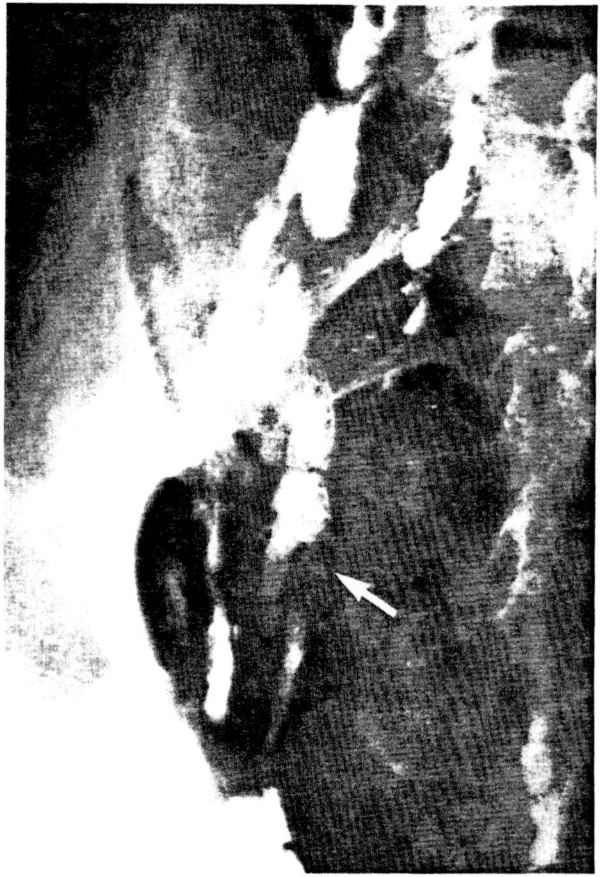

Figure 13a. Teratoma of testis: original lymphogram regarded as probably normal.

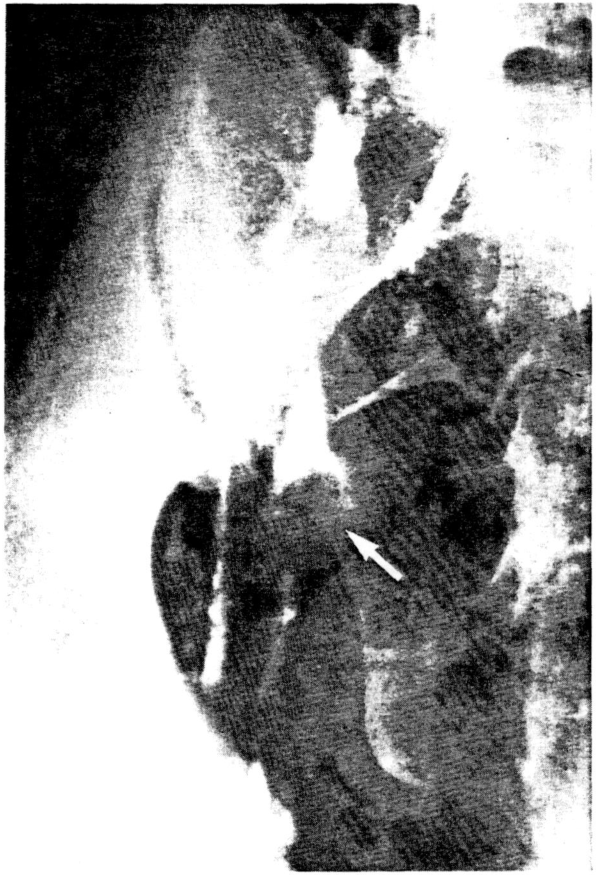

Figure 13b. Subsequent re-examination after six weeks shows obvious metastasis.

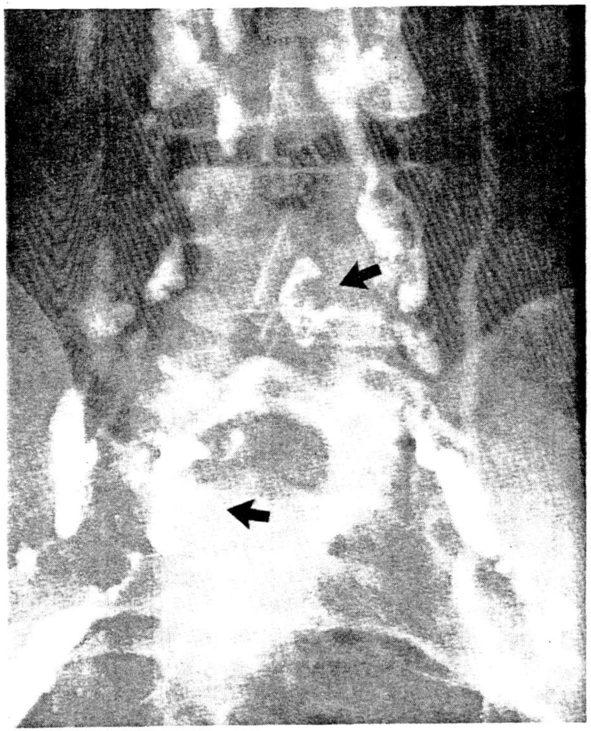

Figure 14a. Carcinoma of cervix: metastatic deposits in two lymph nodes.

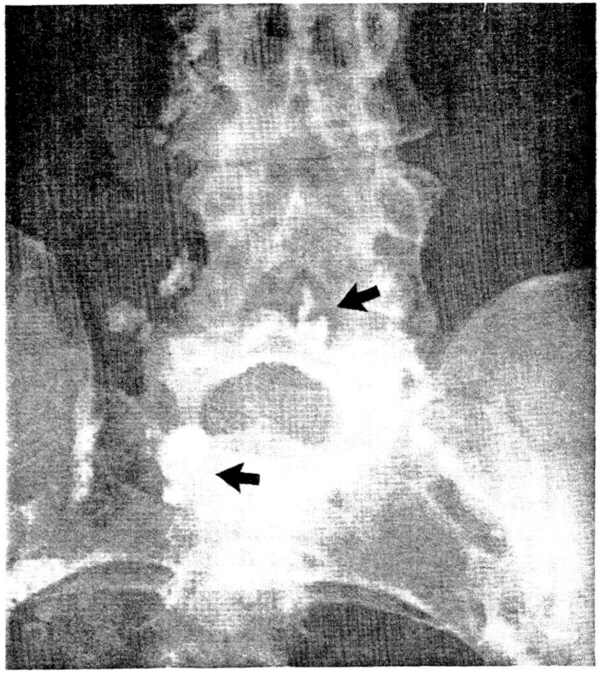

Figure 14b. Shrinkage of deposits after radiotherapy.

Although it has been long accepted for staging of testicular tumours [8, 9] it is similarly true that lymphography fails to detect 20–25% of metastases in such patients [1]. Reasons for failure to demonstrate such deposits include microscopic lesions, non-opacified tumour involved nodes, and lymph nodes completely replaced by tumour. Although staging laparotomy has been carried out for testicular tumours, it has not obtained widespread acceptance.

The availability of new modalities of imaging, including CT and ultrasound, have been widely exploited to attempt to enhance the accuracy of staging in abdominal lymph node disease.

At the present time CT could probably replace abdominal lymphography in the initial staging and follow-up of the patients with lymphoma [20] (Figs. 15a, b). CT has the advantage of being non-invasive and easily repeatable; it is equally satisfactory in those patients in whom lymphography is difficult due to technical problems with the injection, is contra-indicated because of heart disease, lung disease or allergy, or is uninformative due to underfilling of the nodes or to obesity of the patient. The estimation of the size of the affected lymph nodes is also better, allowing more accurate delineation of radiotherapy fields, and facilitating computer-based radiotherapy field planning. In addition to detecting lymphadenopathy in anatomical areas where lymphography is uninformative, CT can on occasion be valuable in the assessment of the liver and spleen. The size of these organs is readily assessed and volume determinations may be made. The presence of tumour deposits may be detected. CT cannot of course be expected to detect lymph node involvement when this is at a microscopic level, and nodes need to be at least 1.5 cm in diameter before significant enlargement may be recognised. Nodes in certain areas such as the retrocrural or upper left para-aortic regions may be suspicious even when they are less than 1.5 cm in diameter since normal nodes in these regions are very small [20]. Thus, although the detection of abdominal lymph node disease by CT is substantially better than that achieved by lymphography, CT is not a substitute for laparotomy if accurate intra-abdominal staging is to be achieved [20]. It is, however, reassuring to note that the incidence of false positive CT examinations is small [20].

CT is also proving more effective than lymphography in the staging and management of testicular tumours [1, 21]. Not only is there an improvement in the detection rate of metastases, but the planning of radiotherapy treatment fields is greatly facilitated. CT is obviously of great value in the monitoring of response to treatment in view of the reproducibility and the non-invasive nature of the technique. Accurate measurements of lymph node size may be made and correlated with the treatment regime in use at

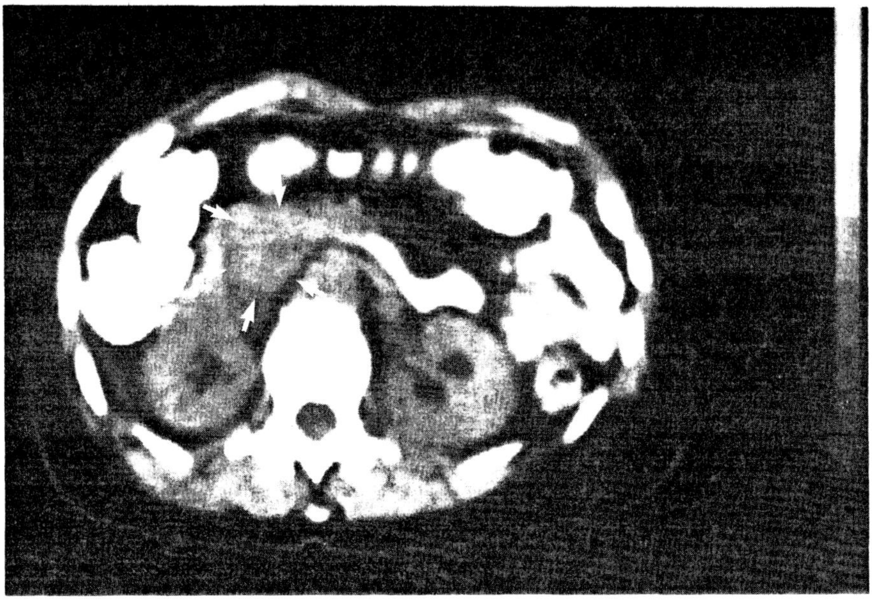

Figure 15a. Hodgkin's disease: CT shows mass of enlarged lymph nodes medial and anterior to the upper pole of the R. kidney (lymphogram technically unsuccessful).

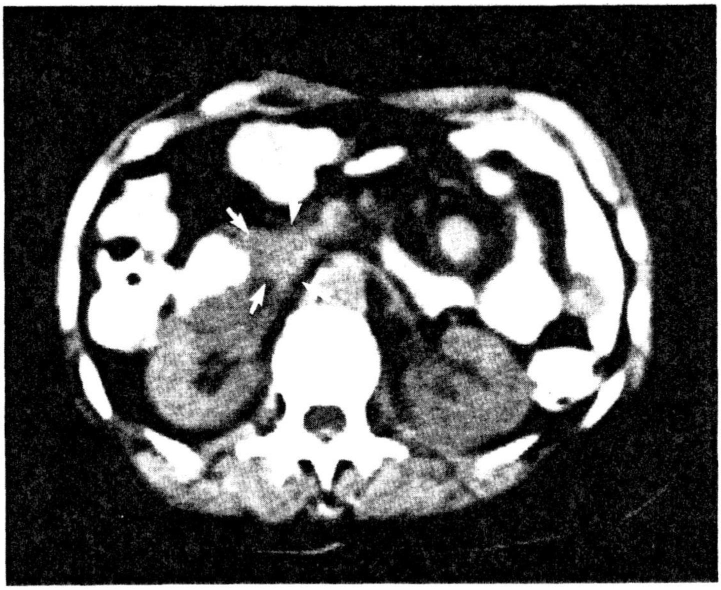

Figure 15b. Same patient: shrinkage of tumour after treatment.

the time. Response to treatment is usually accompanied by shrinkage of the affected nodes, though on occasion cystic changes occur and may cause the node to fail to shrink or even to enlarge. This occurrence may be recognised on CT.

The place of ultra-sonography is more difficult to evaluate at the present time in view of the continuing improvement of available apparatus. There are inherent limitations in the use of ultrasound since the areas of anatomical interest may be obscured by intestinal gas and obesity may prevent adequate ultrasound examination. In addition the technique is highly operator dependent. Nevertheless, there have been a number of reports of the value of ultrasound in assessing abdominal lymph node enlargement [22, 23]. Abdominal lymph nodes enlarged by tumour metastases or lymphoma deposits generally show enlargement with an almost trans-sonic appearance (Fig. 16). Response to treatment may be accompanied by shrinkage and by increased echogenicity. Occasionally treated nodes may fail to shrink but may become cystic and therefore trans-sonic. Lymphadenopathy may be detected in those areas where the nodes are unopacified by lymphography (Fig. 17). The present state of knowledge would suggest that although ultra-sonography has a part to play in the assessment of abdominal lymph node disease, it is unlikely that the accuracy will ever be as high as that achieved by CT. It is, however, cheaper and more widely available than CT.

In those cases where lymph node enlargement is demonstrated by ultrasound, it is possible to follow the progress of the lesion after treatment on serial examination (Figs. 18a, b).

Tumour seeking agents, particularly gallium 67, are of value in the detection of abdominal lymph node disease, particularly in the lymphomas [2]. Gallium 67 scanning is particularly of value in the detection of disease in the upper abdominal and retrocrural lymph nodes. The assessment of gallium 67 abdominal scans is complicated by the accumulation of the isotope in the gastro-intestinal tract, and it is therefore important that the bowel be cleared if possible before the scans are obtained.

The three main modalities of lymph node imaging, i.e. lymphography, CT, and ultrasound, all offer an opportunity for percutaneous biopsy of suspicious lymph nodes. The lymph node is identified by one or other of these techniques and tissue for cytology is obtained by passing a fine (22 gauge) needle percutaneously. CT scanner attachments and suitable ultrasound probes are available for the control of the course of the needle, and the position of the tip is confirmed during the examination. The tissue obtained, however, is only suitable for cytological diagnosis which may be of limited value, particularly in the case of the lymphomas. Histological

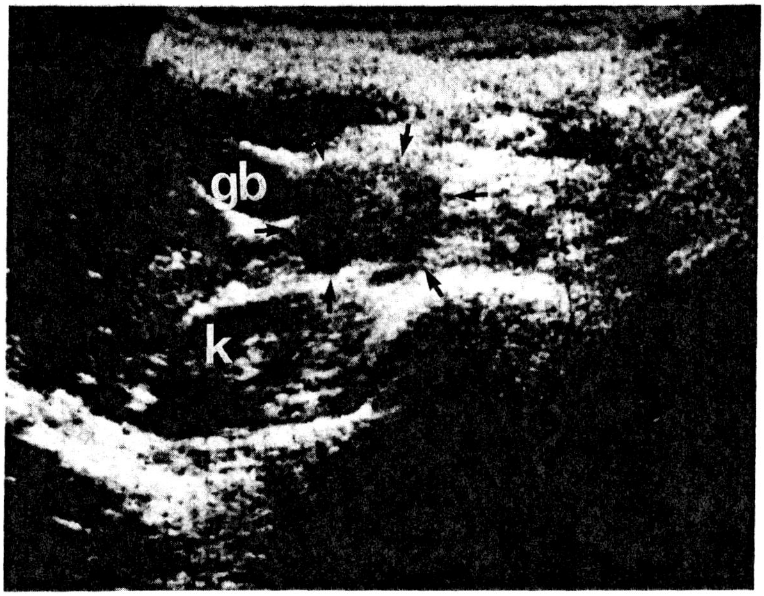

Figure 16. Ultrasound scan of upper abdomen showing lymph node deposits: Hodgkin's disease. (gb-gall bladder; k-kidney).

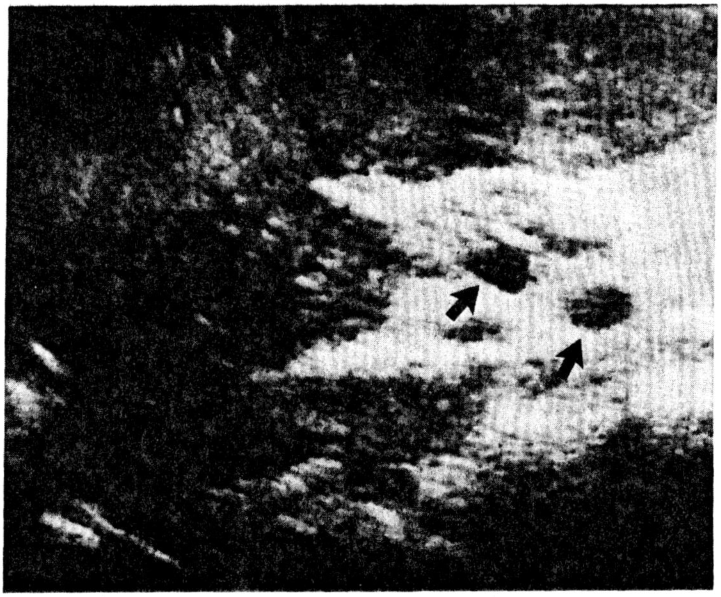

Figure 17. Sagittal ultrasound scan of upper abdomen. Lymph node enlargement in the region of the coeliac axis: Hodgkin's disease.

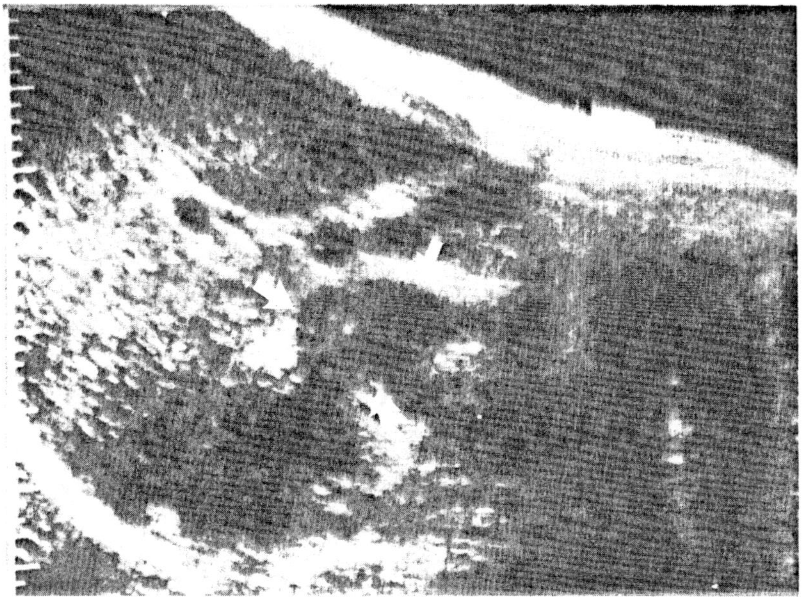

Figure 18a. Lymph node mass in patient with a testicular teratoma. Parasagittal ultrasound scan of upper abdomen shows tumour anterior and medial to R. kidney.

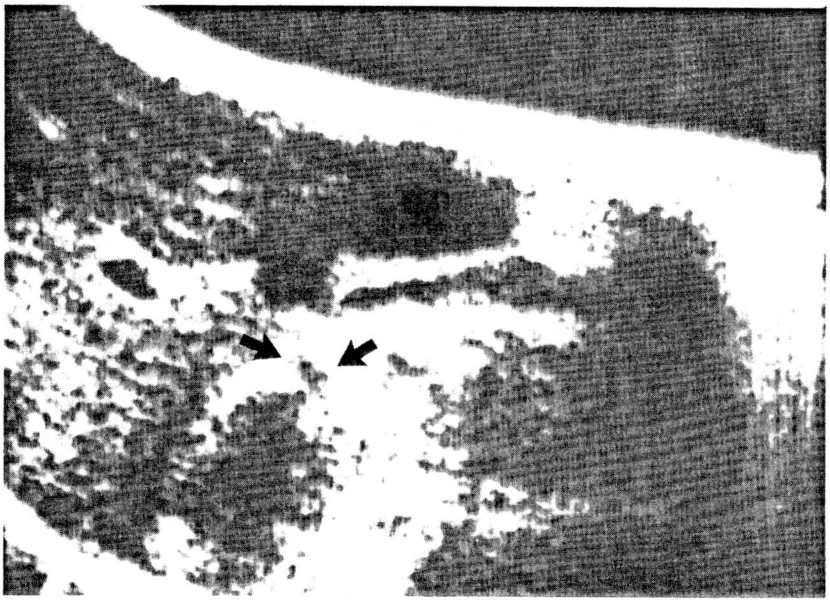

Figure 18b. Marked shrinkage of mass after chemotherapy.

difficulties may also result from the presence of reactive changes due to lipiodol following lymphography. Nevertheless, guided needle biopsy may well come to play an important part in the management and follow-up of patients with intra-abdominal malignancy and in the assessment of the response to treatment [24].

5. Uterus and ovary

The assessment of secondary spread from tumours of the uterus and ovary is partly dealt with in those sections above relating to the lung and to the abdominal lymph nodes. The assessment of primary tumours of the female pelvic organs is at present for the most part carried out by clinical examination, laparoscopy, and the histological study of curettings and other biopsy material. The services of the imaging department are not often required.

Conventional radiography has a limited part to play, mainly in the assessment of the secondary effects of primary tumours of the uterus and ovary on the adjacent urinary tract organs and bowel (Figs. 19, 20). Angiography has been used for the assessment of trophoblastic tumours of the uterus as they are lesions of great vascularity whose extent is well shown on angiographic studies (Fig. 21). Extra-uterine deposits may be visualised in addition to the primary tumour in the uterus (Fig. 22). However, the contribution of such studies to the management of the disease is questionable and angiography is not widely practised for this purpose, particularly as the patients are young and minimisation of radiation exposure is important.

Ultrasonography is often used for the assessment of trophoblastic tumours [25]. These lesions show a vesicular pattern with sonolucent areas surrounded by high intensity echoes (Fig. 23). Myometrial invasion cannot readily be recognised. The uterine tumour volume may be determined by ultrasound and correlated with the level of human chorionic gonadotrophin (HCG). Theca lutein cysts may also be detected and measured. Ultrasound is complementary to serum HCG levels in the follow-up and treatment of trophoblastic disease and in the detection of persistent trophoblastic disease. Ultrasound examination has the advantage of being non-invasive and therefore readily repeatable, an important aspect of the management of a curable tumour affecting women of childbearing age.

It is possible to demonstrate pelvic anatomy in great detail by the use of CT, which may therefore be used for the staging of tumours and in the planning of their treatment [26, 27]. In particular, spread of the tumour laterally towards the pelvic walls is detectable in situations where a full

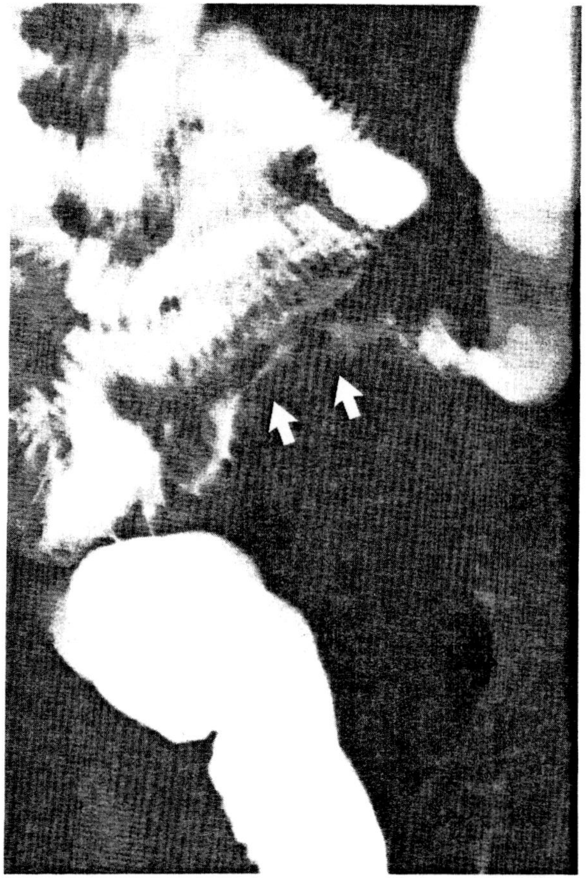

Figure 19. Barium enema in patient with ovarian carcinoma showing extrinsic compression and invasion of sigmoid colon.

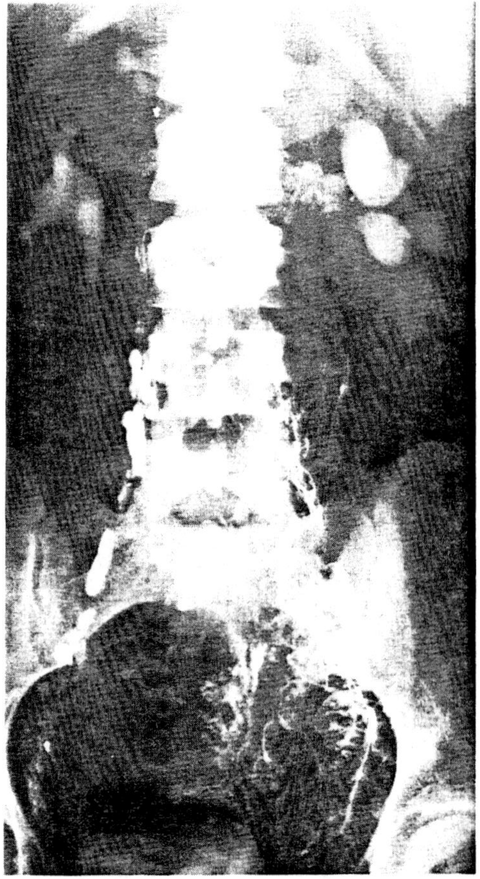

Figure 20. I.V.P. in patient with advanced carcinoma of the cervix showing L. hydronephrosis and hydro-ureter. Note extensive collateral lymphatic circulation due to obstruction.

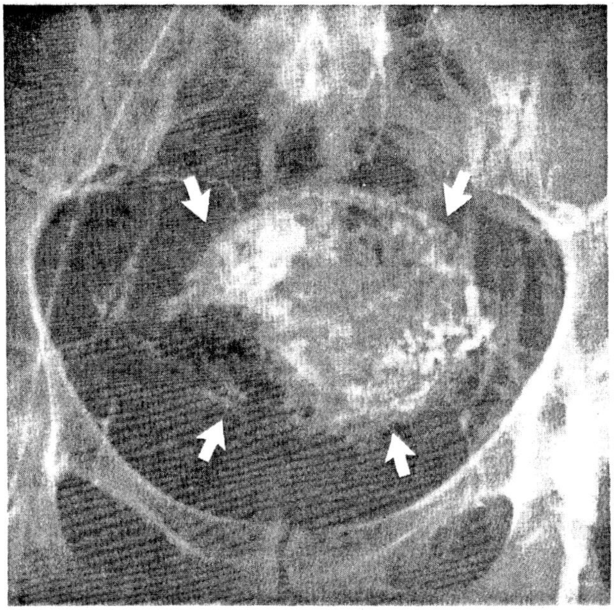

Figure 21. Choriocarcinoma: angiogram shows extensive tumour circulation.

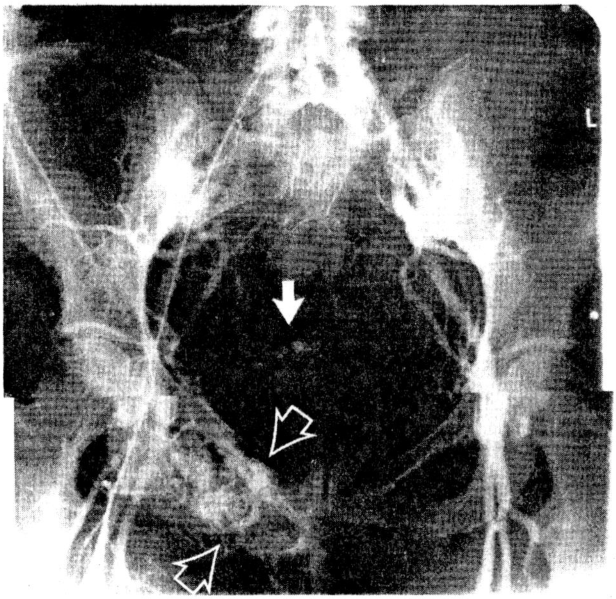

Figure 22. Choriocarcinoma: angiogram shows minimal residual uterine tumour after curettage (↙), but a large paravaginal deposit (⇩).

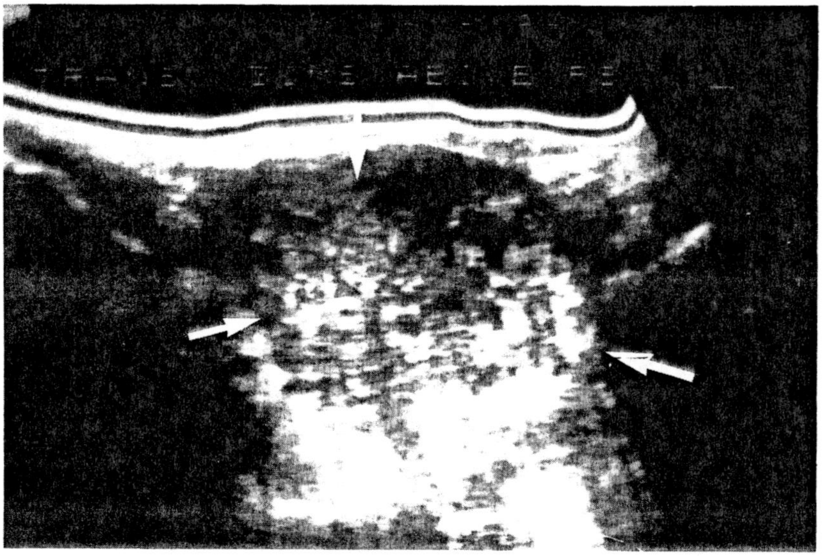

Figure 23. Trophoblastic tumour: ultrasound scan of uterus showing complex vesicular mass.

clinical appraisal may be difficult. The influence of the use of such techniques on the prognosis has yet to be evaluated.

6. Testis

The staging and follow up of testicular tumours is related to the detection of metastatic spread particularly to the abdominal lymph nodes and to the lungs as described above.

7. Urinary tract

Although many tumours of the urinary tract are diagnosed by imaging methods, the management of most tumours, particularly those of the kidney and ureter, is surgical and imaging is largely irrelevant in follow-up of the primary tumour, though it may play a part in the management of its more distant spread. As in the case of the uterine tumours, the staging of prostatic and bladder tumours may be enhanced by the use of CT [28, 29] but its value in the management of these tumours has yet to be evaluated fully. Similarly the role of ultrasound imaging in bladder and prostatic tumour is not yet fully established. The secondary spread of urinary tract tumours to the abdominal lymph nodes may be assessed as indicated above, by lymphography, CT and ultrasound.

Imaging of the urinary tract is of great value where it is involved secondarily by malignant disease and its role in the assessment of the response to treatment is therefore particularly evident in the demonstration of any regression of recurrence of obstructive changes (Figs. 24a, b). Intravenous urography is of value both in the assessment of renal function as well as renal anatomy, but is ineffective where obstruction has caused the kidney to become non-functioning. In this clinical situation ultrasound examination may be of great value (Fig. 25), and the same abnormalities may also be demonstrated by CT. Mass lesions may occur in the kidneys in the lymphomas and may be detected by intravenous urography and by ultrasound (Fig. 26). As in the case of lymph nodes, lymphoma deposits in the kidneys have a transonic appearance.

Renography using ^{131}I hippuran or some similar agent is a useful and non-invasive method of assessing renal function. Obstructive uropathy may be readily diagnosed and objective measurements of renal function may be made allowing accurate assessment of the response to treatment.

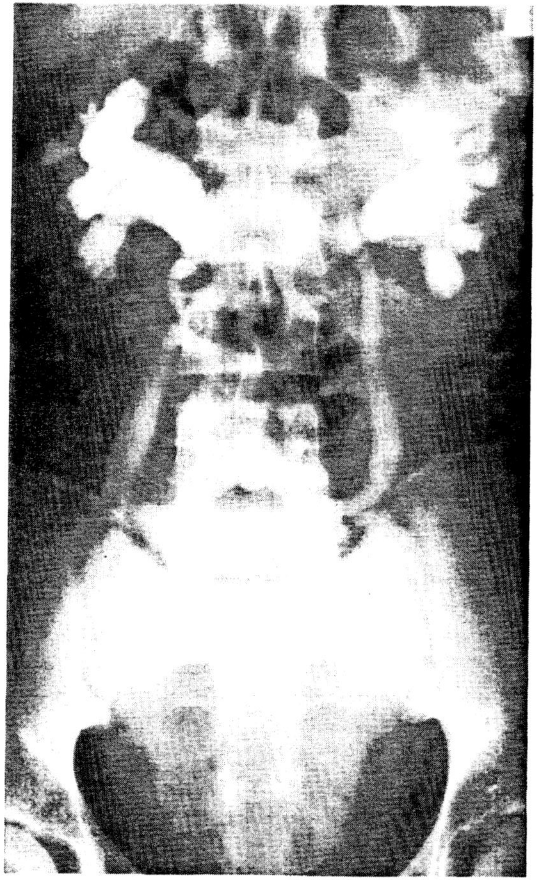

Figure 24a. **Advanced tumour of the ovary (dysgerminoma):** bilateral hydronephrosis.

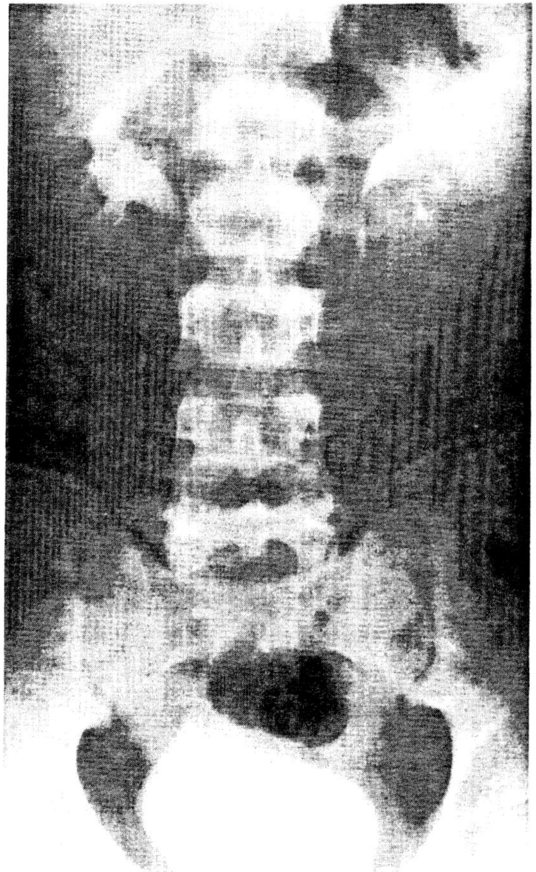

Figure 24b. **Marked improvement after radiotherapy.** Residual deformity of bladder.

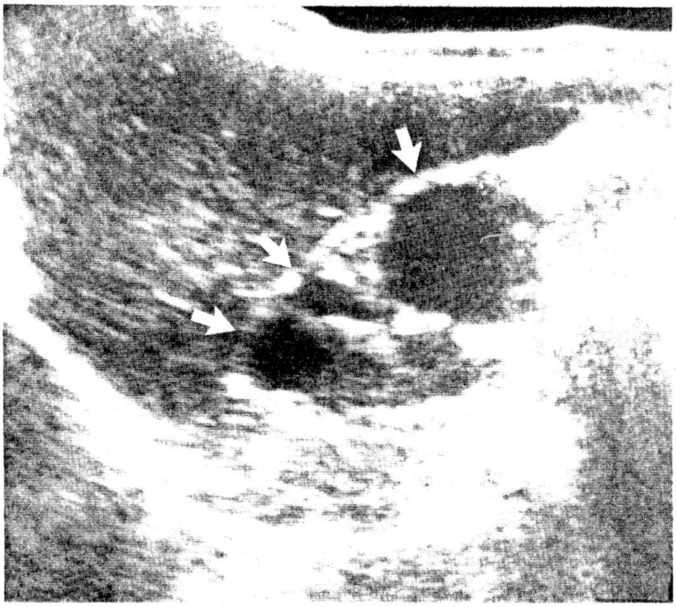

Figure 25. **Ultrasound examination of 'nonfunctioning kidney' shows marked hydronephrosis.**

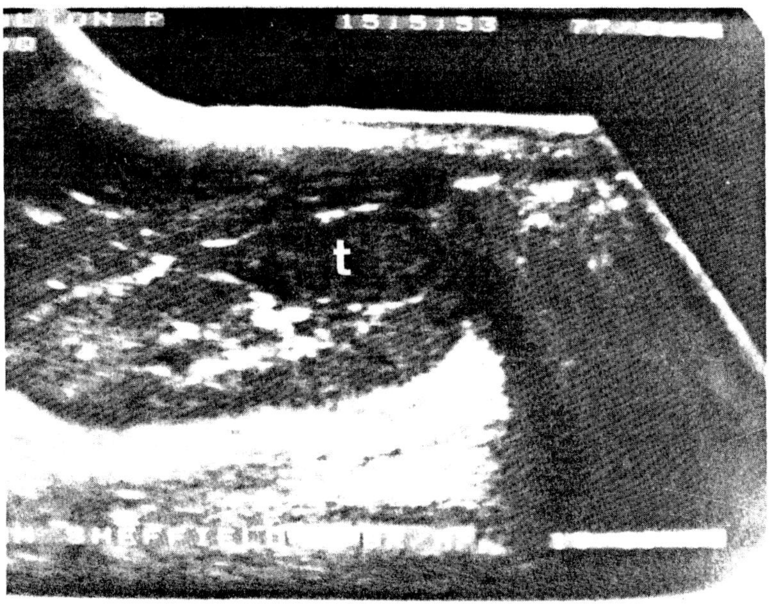

Figure 26. **Hodgkin's deposit in kidney shown by ultrasound (t).**

8. Thyroid

Conventional radiological techniques have a limited role in the imaging of thyroid tumours; benign and malignant tumours may simply be of soft tissue density. Benign adenomata commonly show dense circumscribed amorphous masses of calcification. The presence of this type of calcification, however, does not in any way exclude malignancy. Malignant lesions sometimes show fine particulate calcifications, most commonly found in papillary carcinomata [30]. Low kilovoltage, high definition radiographic technique is necessary to show this type of abnormality.

Compression of the trachea is commonly found in thyroid tumours; actual invasion is only seen in association with malignant tumours, and is better evaluated in tomograms than on plain radiographs. Invasion of the oesophagus occurs less frequently.

Thyroid tumours commonly metastasise particularly to the lung (see section 1) and to bone (see section 8). Lung deposits are most often discrete, rounded lesions which may become very large ('cannonball' metastases). Occasionally miliary deposits are seen evenly distributed through the lungs [31], and may be less easy to detect (Fig. 27). Bone deposits occur most frequently in the ribs, spine and pelvis and are almost invariably osteolytic.

The thyroid was one of the first organs to be imaged using radioactive isotopes, because of the physiological avidity of thyroid tissue for iodine. The ^{131}I and ^{125}I isotopes may be used, or alternatively technetium 99m (as sodium pertechnate), which is taken up by the thyroid in a manner similar to iodine. The uptake of isotope may be used both for imaging and function studies. Thyroid tumour tissue generally shows a lower isotope uptake than normal thyroid, and a tumour therefore appears as a 'cold' region on a thyroid scan. This cannot be distinguished from a cold area due to an adenoma, cyst or haemorrhage. The uptake of isotope in the tumour is small because of the greater avidity of the normal thyroid tissue, and metastases cannot therefore be imaged in most cases unless the normal thyroid tissue is either ablated using radio-active iodine or is surgically removed. The same constraints apply to the treatment of thyroid tumour metastases by radioactive iodine, which will not accumulate in the metastases in sufficient concentration in the presence of normally active thyroid tissue. Following ablation or thyroidectomy, tumour metastases may be readily imaged, the uptake of isotope depending on the degree of differentiation of the tumour. Metastases, as indicated above are most often found in bone and lung tissue (Fig. 28), but may also be found in the mediastinum, and in the brain. The information obtained is useful not only from a diagnostic point of view, but

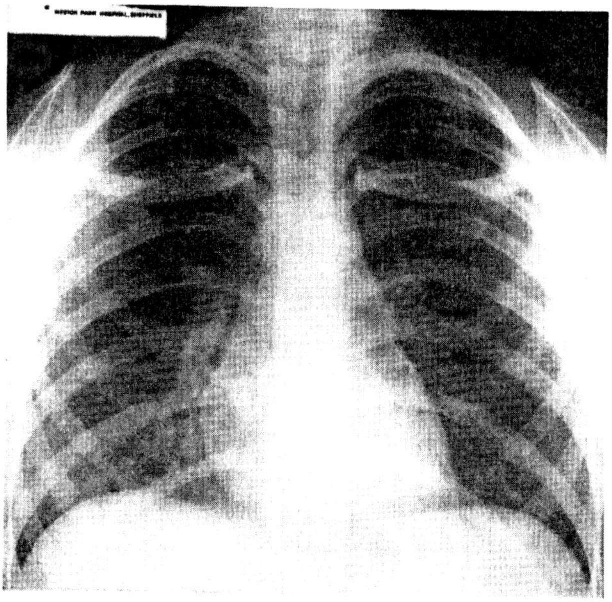

Figure 27. Carcinoma of thyroid, recurrent after radical surgery: widespread fine pulmonary nodulation.

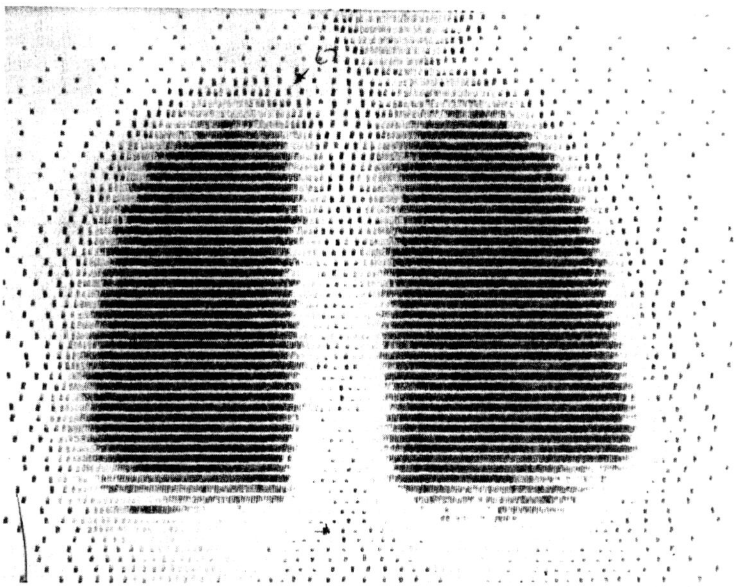

Figure 28. Iodine 131 scan: diffuse pulmonary uptake of isotope (same patient as Fig. 27).

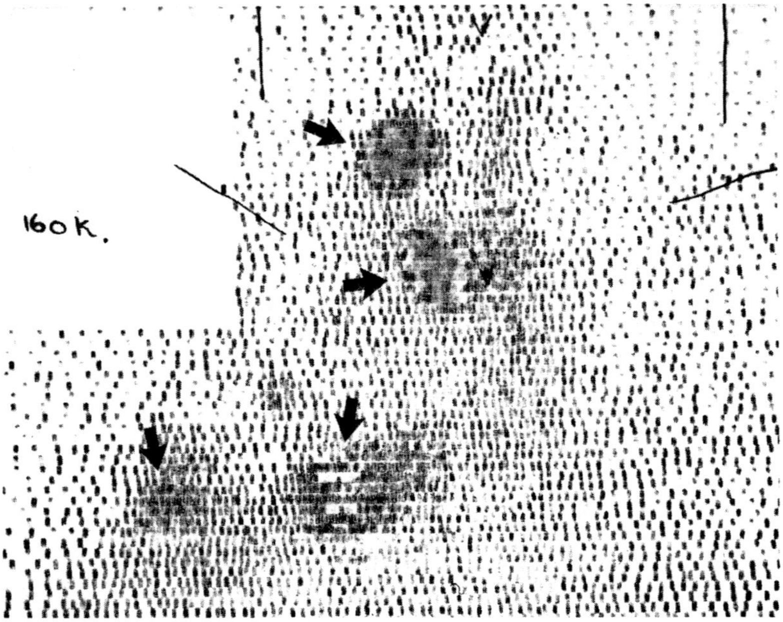

Figure 29a. Iodine 131 scan: lymph node metastases in neck and supraclavicular fossa.

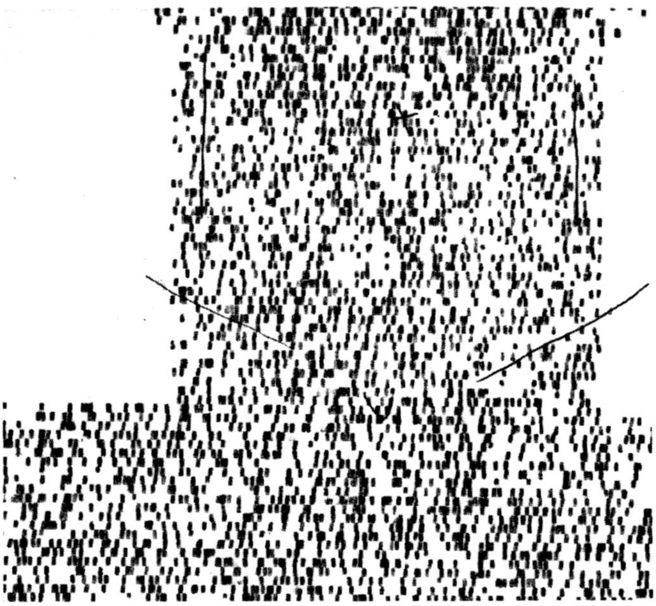

Figure 29b. After ablation no uptake seen.

also to assess the potential for isotope ablation of the secondary deposits. Ablation may be confirmed by the disappearance of the previously demonstrated areas of isotope uptake on subsequent scans (Figs. 29a, b).

9. Bones

The assessment of bone tumours and their progress is generally carried out both by conventional radiological methods and by radio-isotope imaging [32]. Primary bone tumours are relatively uncommon. The radiographic changes include a mass associated with bone destruction, reactive new bone formation and tumour calcification or new bone formation. Response is indicated by a reduction in the volume of any mass present, together with repair and sclerosis of destroyed and infiltrated bone (Figs. 30a, b). Bone seeking isotopes are often taken up by primary bone tumours and the reparative processes following treatment will result in a reduction in uptake [33]. Normal bone included in the field will also show a reduction in isotope uptake not necessarily associated with any radiological changes. Pulmonary and hepatic metastases from osteosarcomas may also show isotope uptake [32]. The fluorine 18 scan is more sensitive than conventional radiology in the early detection of lung deposits from an osteosarcoma [34]. In some situations CT may be of value in the management of primary bone tumours and in the assessment of response to treatment. In particular the extra-osseous component of the tumour is very well shown.

Secondary bone tumours are considerably more common than primary tumours. A major proportion arise from primary tumours of the breast and bronchus because of the high incidence of such tumours and the frequent occurrence of bone metastasis. However, primary tumours in the prostate, thyroid and kidney also cause bone metastases, and with varying frequency most tumours may be associated with bony metastases. Multifocal bone deposits are also seen in multiple myelomatosis. Depending on the primary tumour and the individual response of the patient, bone metastases may produce either lytic or sclerotic changes in the affected bones, or a combination of the two. In those cases producing bone lysis, response to treatment is often accompanied by sclerosis in the affected areas, though on occasion anatomical repair will occur with relatively little sclerosis or other bony deformity (Figs. 31a, b). In those cases where the bone reaction is sclerotic there is a variable response. Sometimes clinical remission is not accompanied by any significant alteration in the pattern of bone lesions, but on occasion the bone sclerosis will diminish with restoration to a more normal

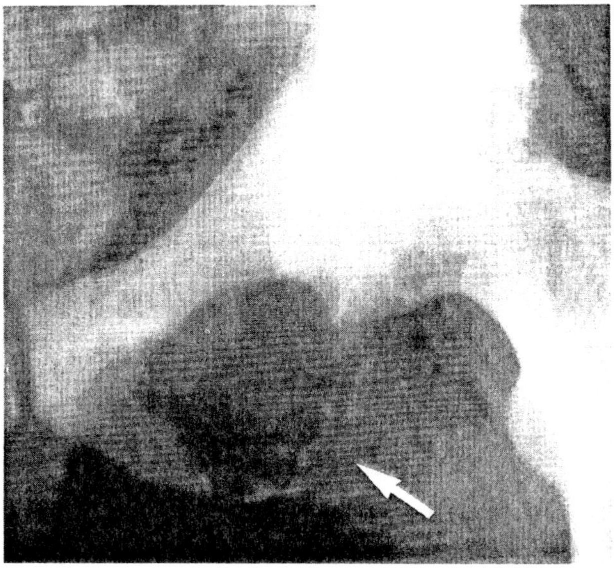

Figure 30a. Paget's disease of bone: osteosarcoma.

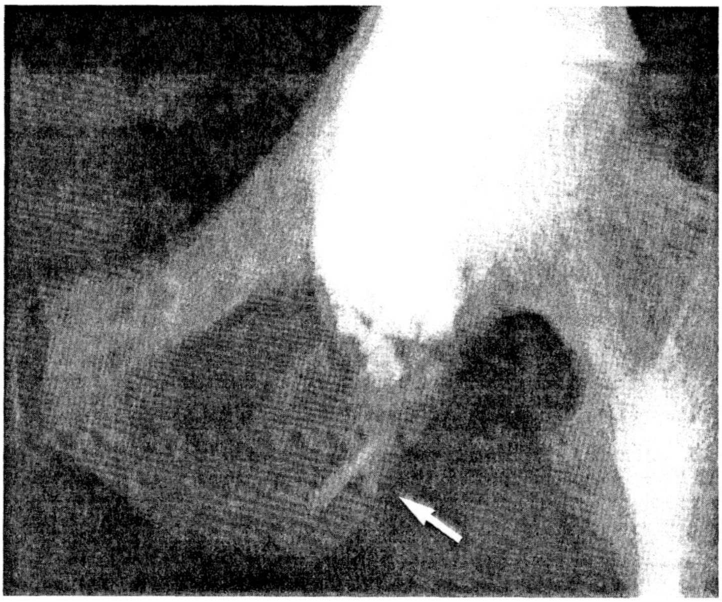

Figure 30b. Repair following radiotherapy.

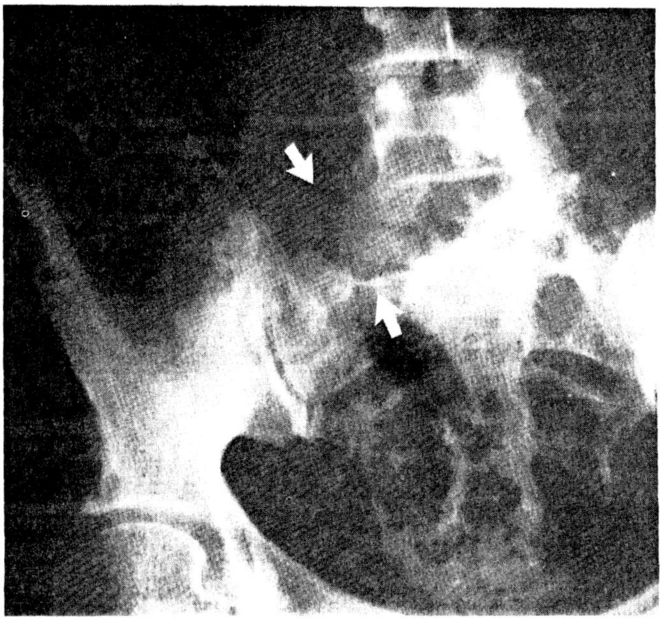

Figure 31a. Carcinoma of breast: large osteolytic metastasis.

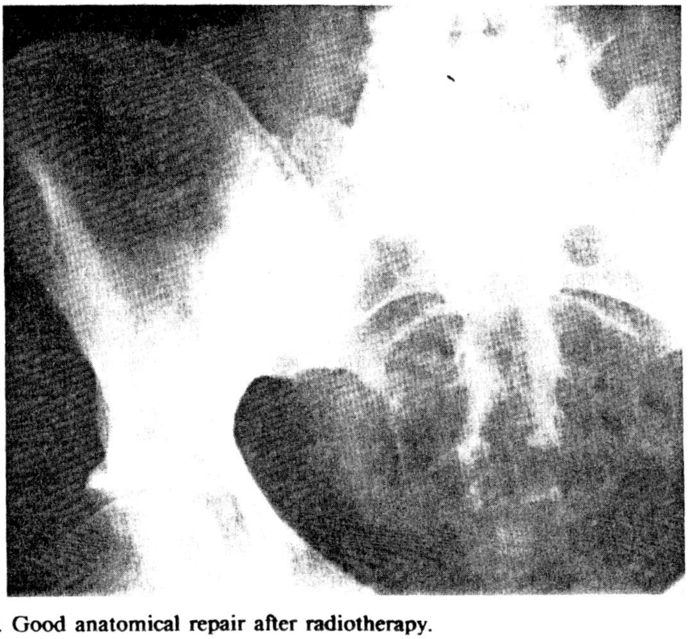

Figure 31b. Good anatomical repair after radiotherapy.

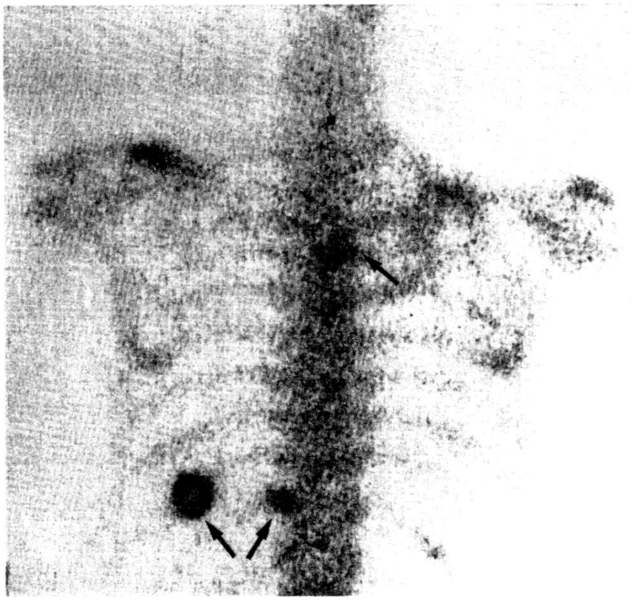

Figure 32. **Technetium 99m diphosphonate bone scan: multiple areas of raised uptake** due to metastases from a carcinoma of breast.

architecture. Myeloma deposits are almost invariably lytic when first seen, but may become sclerotic after treatment.

Bone metastases may be readily overlooked on radiological examination, particularly when they lie in cancellous bone [35]. Radio-isotope imaging will detect metastatic bone tumours before they are visible radiologically [32]. In prostatic carcinoma, for example, radio-isotope imaging may reveal the presence of metastases for up to 3 years before they become radiologically visible [32]. Metastases appear as localised areas of high isotope uptake (Fig. 32) and response to treatment may be accompanied by a diminution or disappearance of the affected area. Initially there may, however, be increased isotope uptake due to repair, particularly in those cases treated by chemotherapy. In breast cancer, abnormal bone scans may return to normal following endocrine therapy [36]. Myeloma deposits, since they produce little or no reactive changes in the surrounding bone, may be unaccompanied by any localised area of isotope uptake. Where there is diffuse skeletal involvement as is sometimes the case in prostatic carcinoma, the increased uptake of radio-isotope may be overlooked because of its diffuse nature [32]. It is generally advisable to obtain radiographs of areas shown to be abnormal on isotope examinations, particularly in the elderly, since areas of high uptake may not necessarily be due to metastatic disease but may turn out to be the result of localised Paget's disease or osteoarthritis, or even fractures.

Lymphoma deposits in bone may be detected by conventional bone scanning agents which may demonstrate metastases before they are radiologically visible [37]. Lymphomatous deposits may also be demonstrated in bone by the use of gallium 67 [2]. Similarly, deposits from a thyroid carcinoma may be imaged by thyroid seeking agents such as iodine 131. Bone metastases are readily demonstrated by CT particularly when they are sclerotic in type [3]. However, because of the multiplicity of tomographic sections necessary to image the whole area of interest, CT scanning is of limited practical value in the detection of bone metastases.

10. Nasal sinuses and nasopharynx

Tumours in this region consist of soft tissue masses often accompanied by bone destruction. The destructive changes are particularly evident in tumours affecting the parasanal sinuses and nasal cavity. The maxillary sinuses are most frequently affected. Nasopharyngeal tumours may be accompanied by bone sclerosis in the base of the skull. Tomography is of value for more detailed evaluation of the extent of any tumour together with any accompanying bone destruction. CT is of particular importance in this area in the accurate anatomical depiction of the site and size of tumour and accompanying bone destruction. Response to treatment is evident as a shrinkage of soft tissue tumour, bone repair, and re-aeration of affected sinuses (Figs. 33a, b). All these effects may be partial and repeated examinations to evaluate response to treatment and the possibility of recurrence are often difficult to assess because of the failure to restore anatomical normality.

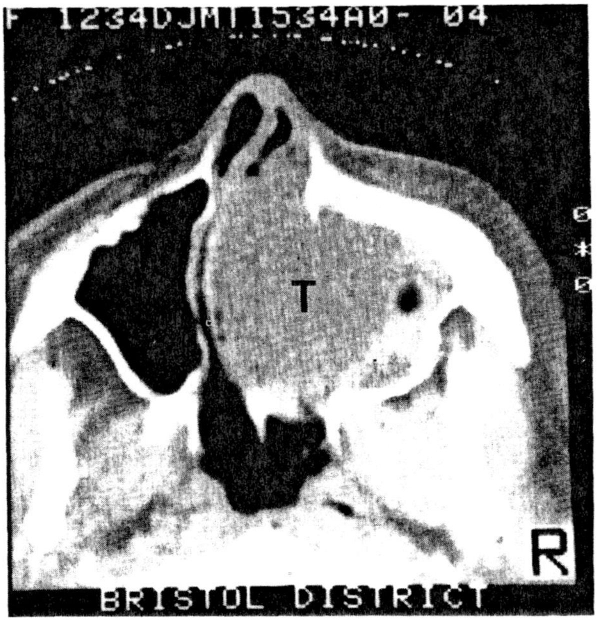

Figure 33a. CT scan: large carcinoma of R. maxillary sinus (T) invading the nasal cavity (courtesy of Dr. F.G.M. Ross, Bristol Royal Infirmary).

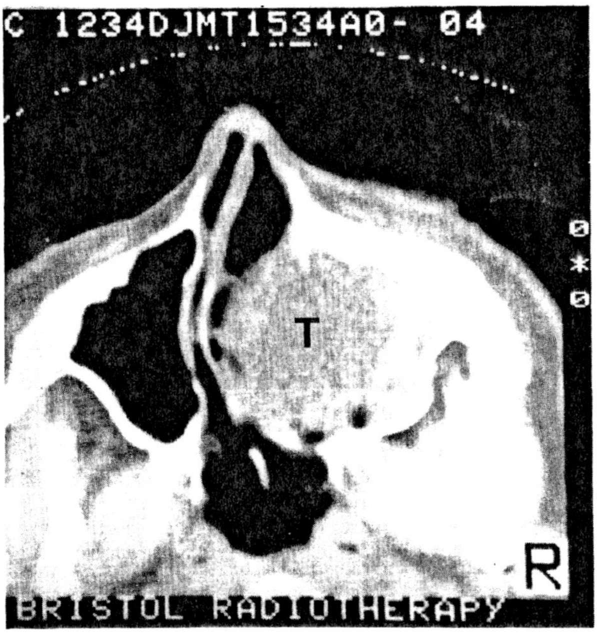

Figure 33b. Shrinkage of tumour after radiotherapy.

11. Larynx

The place of imaging in the management of tumours of the larynx is limited. Until recently it was true to say that the role of radiology was largely confined to the assessment of subglottic spread of laryngeal tumours. The glottic and supraglottic portions of such tumours could generally be visualised by direct inspection. More recently, however, the role of CT in the three dimensional assessment of laryngeal tumours has been reported [38] and it may well prove to have a place in the pre-treatment assessment of such tumours and the monitoring of the results of treatment.

There is still, however, a place for conventional methods, including tomography and laryngography. Both techniques are capable of demonstrating the extent of laryngeal tumours, including any subglottic spread, and may be used in the assessment of response to treatment (Figs. 34, 35).

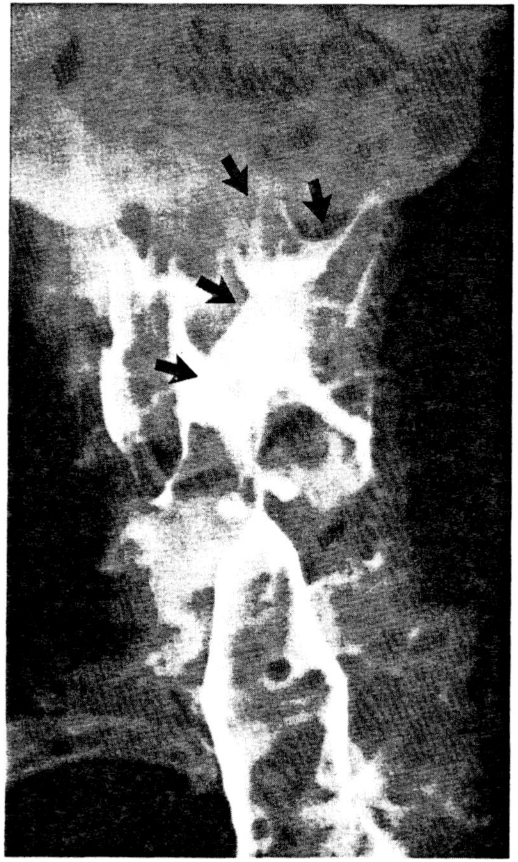

Figure 34. Laryngogram: supraglottic carcinoma of larynx.

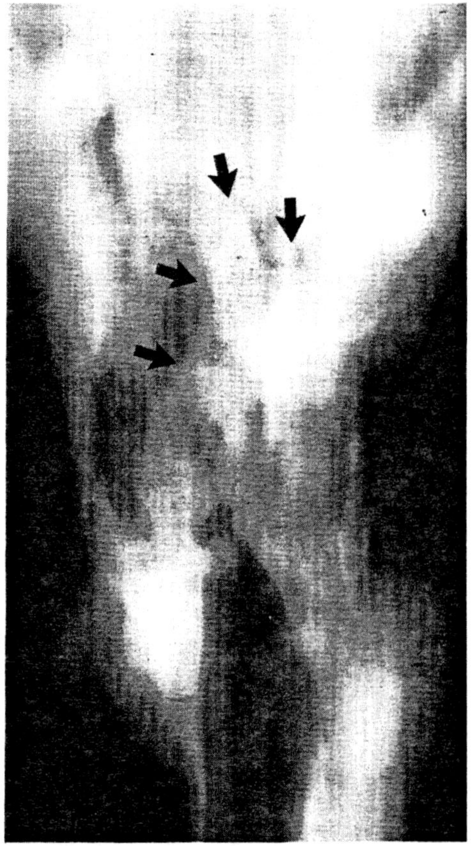

Figure 35. Tomogram of same patient as Fig. 34.

12. Gastro-intestinal tract

The gastro-intestinal tract is usually examined by outlining it with barium sulphate. CT has a limited part to play in the assessment and monitoring of abdominal tumours arising from or affecting the tract. The oesophagus, stomach and intestines may all be affected both by primary tumours and by extrinsic compression and invasion (Fig. 36). Strictures and deformities are usually recognisable as being either intrinsic or extrinsic. In those cases not managed by surgical means radiological observation of the progress following treatment may be useful (Figs. 37a, b). Dysphagia following treatment of an oseophageal tumour is common and may be caused by oesophagitis following radiotherapy, peptic oesophagitis, monilia or as well as the more obvious possibility of recurrent tumour. Radiological distinction of these abnormalities is usually possible. Primary tumours of the stomach and intestine are for the most part outside the scope of this discussion. Lymphomatous invasion of the stomach or intestine may occur both as a manifestation of primary extra-nodal lymphoma and as a complication of pre-existing lymphomatous disease. Such lesions may appear as strictures, mural infiltration, intra-luminal and extra-luminal masses, and as ulcerative lesions. Radiological assessment and follow-up may be of value (Figs. 38a, b).

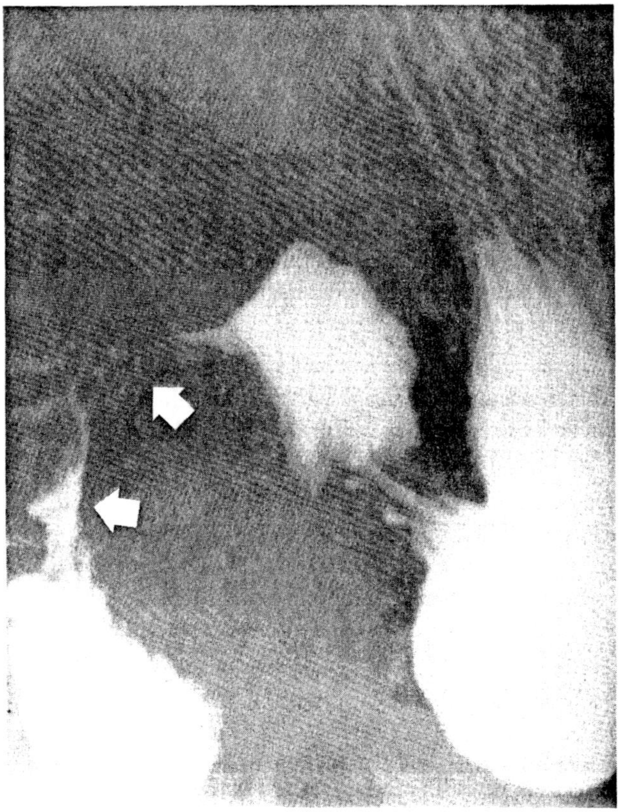

Figure 36. Barium meal: extrinsic compression of duodenum due to metastases from a testicular seminoma.

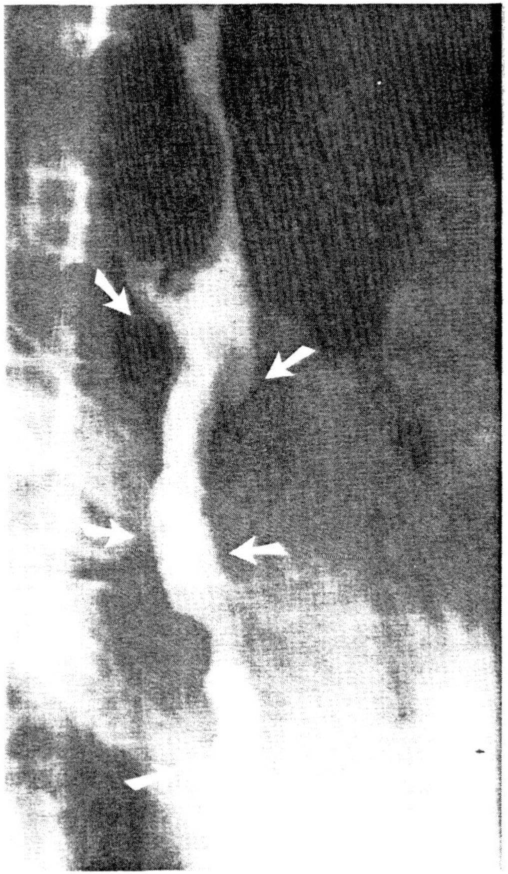

Figure 37a. Barium swallow: carcinoma of the oesophagus.

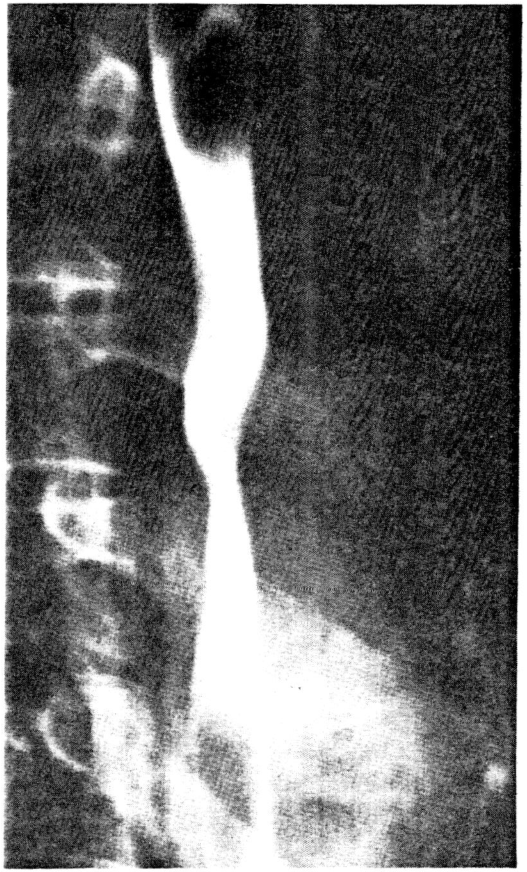

Figure 37b. Stricture much improved after radiotherapy.

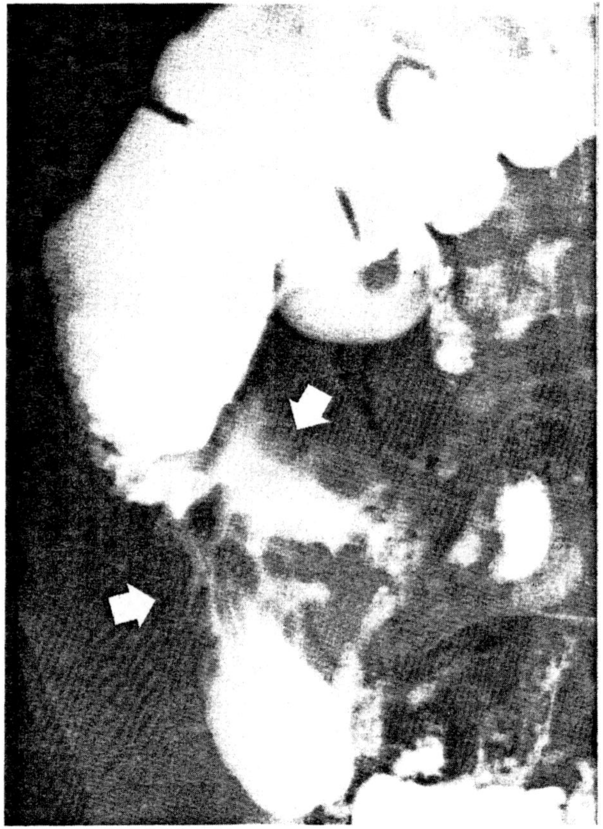

Figure 38a. Lymphoma of caecum shown by barium enema examination.

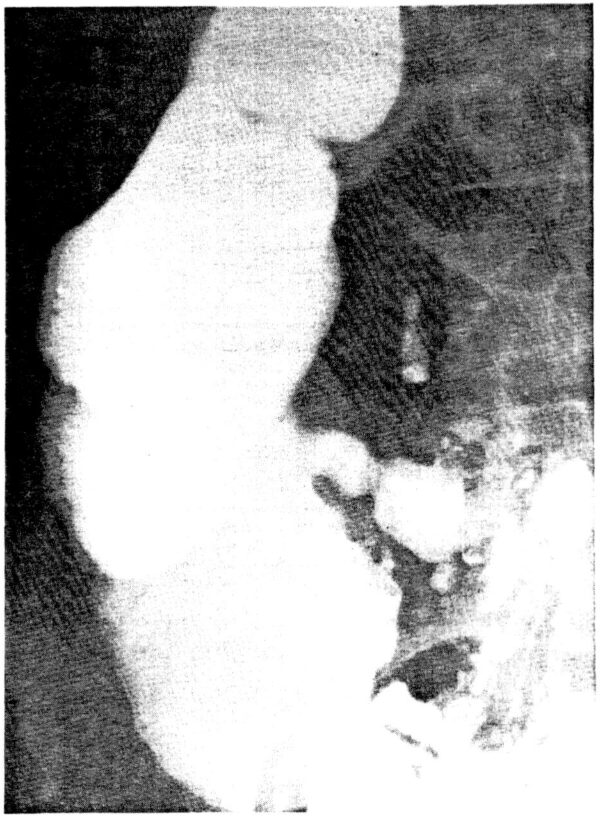

Figure 38b. Disappearance of tumour after chemotherapy.

13. Liver, spleen and pancreas

The numerous ways now available to image these organs are mainly of recent development. The shadows of both liver and spleen appear on plain radiographs of the abdomen and may be of some value for the monitoring of tumour response. The liver and spleen may be readily imaged by radio-isotope methods. Those in most frequent use involve the use of labelled colloids such as Technetium 99m sulphur colloid. Measurement of the size of the liver and spleen may be readily carried out and may be of value in the assessment of response. With a suitable apparatus true volume measurements are possible. It should be noted, however, that enlargement of the spleen may simply be a reactive phenomenon and does not necessarily indicate infiltration. Enlargement of the liver may be diffuse or may be associated with areas of defective radio-isotope uptake due to discrete tumour deposits (Fig. 39). Tumour deposits smaller than 2 cm cannot generally be detected.

Ultrasound examination may be used to demonstrate the size of the liver and can also demonstrate infiltrative or space-occupying lesions of primary or metastatic origin. It is probable that the technique is rather more sensitive than isotope methods for the demonstration of small hepatic metastases and because of the non-invasive nature of the procedure repeated examinations are possible for the monitoring of such lesions. Metastases show a variable appearance on ultrasound examination, some appearing relatively anechoic, whereas others show increased echoes. Complex 'target' and 'bull's eye' metastases are also described (Fig. 40). Meticulous ultrasound scanning will reveal over 90% of metastases exceeding 1 cm in diameter [22]. The volume of discrete deposits may be measured in some cases. Computed tomography will also show hepatic metastases but in some cases they are difficult to detect because their density is so similar to that of the normal liver tissue. Contrast enhancement does not usually improve the density difference to any appreciable degree since both the metastasis and the liver substance both take up the contrast medium. However, in the case of necrotic metastases, contrast enhancement may reveal an increase in density difference.

Assessment of the spleen may be carried out by isotopic or ultrasound techniques. Both diffuse enlargement and discrete deposits may be shown. The size of the spleen may be measured and serial measurements may provide an index of tumour response [39].

Angiography is occasionally carried out for primary liver tumours both as a diagnostic procedure and therapeutically to allow either embolisation or infusion of cytotoxic drugs into the tumour. As such procedures are often

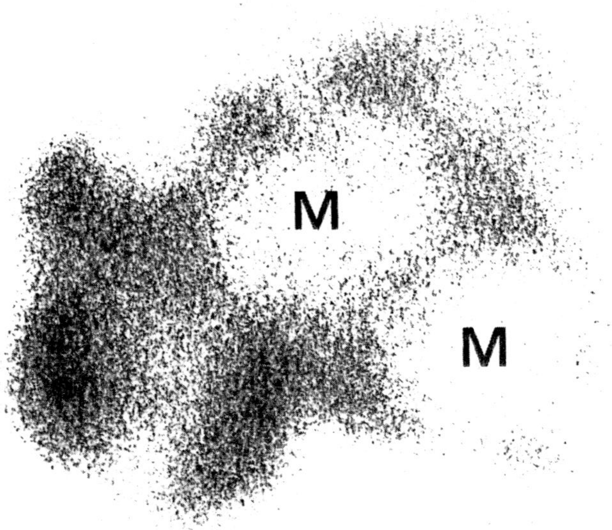

Figure 39. Technetium 99m sulphur colloid liver scan showing large filling defects due to metastases (M) from a carcinoma of the bronchus.

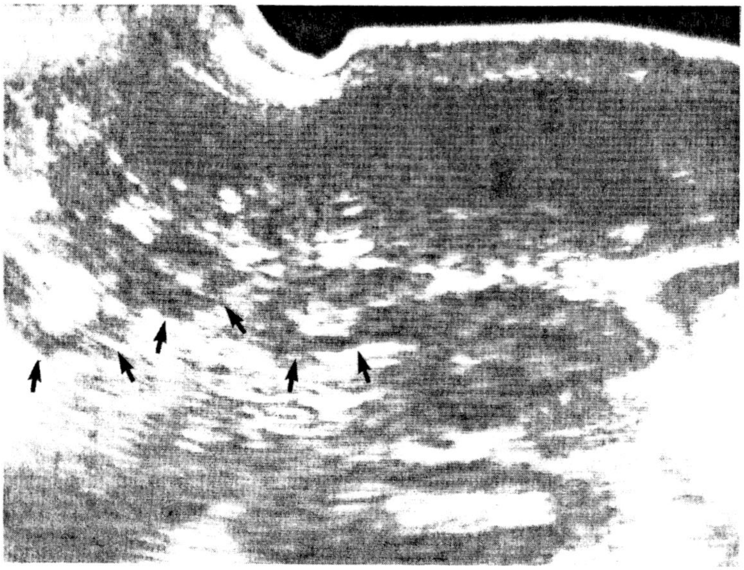

Figure 40. 'Target metastases' in liver shown by ultrasound examination: carcinoma of the colon.

repeated on a number of occasions, the vascularity of the tumour may be observed angiographically on each occasion, and assessment of any response made.

Jaundiced patients may be examined by ultrasound or CT. Both examinations are capable of showing dilated intra-hepatic bile ducts indicating extra-hepatic biliary obstructions. Information as to the site of the obstruction may be derived by percutaneous transhepatic cholangiography. Alternatively, contrast medium may be injected distal to the obstruction by endoscopic catheterisation. This will allow both pancreatic and the common bile ducts to be opacified. Tumours of the pancreas are generally diagnosed either by ultrasound examination or by CT. Where a satisfactory ultrasound examination is possible the accuracy of the techniques is comparable.

14. The central nervous system

Brain tumours, both primary and secondary, are most commonly imaged at the present time by computed tomography. Isotope imaging is a useful alternative in some cases, but is a rather less sensitive technique. In the case of those cerebral tumours not managed by surgical methods, CT is of value in the monitoring of response to treatment (Figs. 41a, b). Some pituitary tumours are managed by non-surgical methods including radiotherapy and drug therapy. In these cases radiological monitoring may be by radiographic examination of the pituitary fossa supplemented by conventional and computed tomography. The latter is of particular value not for the assessment of the intrasellar component of the tumour but for its suprasellar extension (Figs. 42a, b).

Spinal tumours, both primary and secondary, may be detected by myelography. Water-soluble contrast media are now used almost exclusively for this procedure, the older oily media having been largely abandoned. In certain cases, however, they still have advantages as they can be left *in situ* allowing the patient to be re-examined radiologically using the same contrast medium. Thus the relief of a spinal block due to secondary neoplasm may be assessed without re-injection of contrast medium into the patient. This practice would not be adopted in patients having a more extended prognosis since oily contrast media left within the theca may cause adhesive arachnoiditis. CT has a limited role in the detection and follow-up of spinal tumours, either as a single technique or in conjunction with the injection of a water soluble contrast medium such as metrizamide.

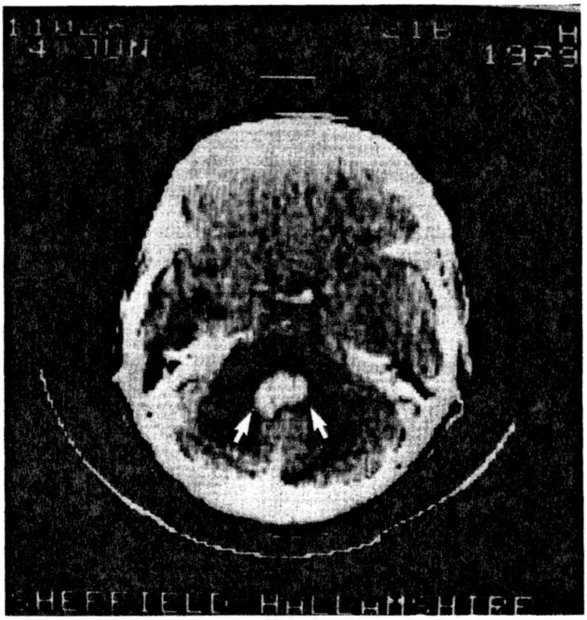

Figure 41a. CT brain scan (contrast enhanced) showing lesion in brain stem: lymphoma deposit.

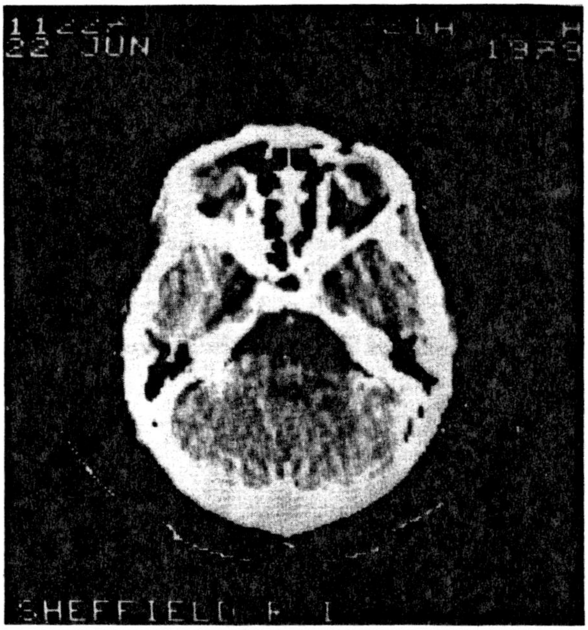

Figure 41b. CT brain scan (enhanced): disappearance of lesion after radiotherapy.

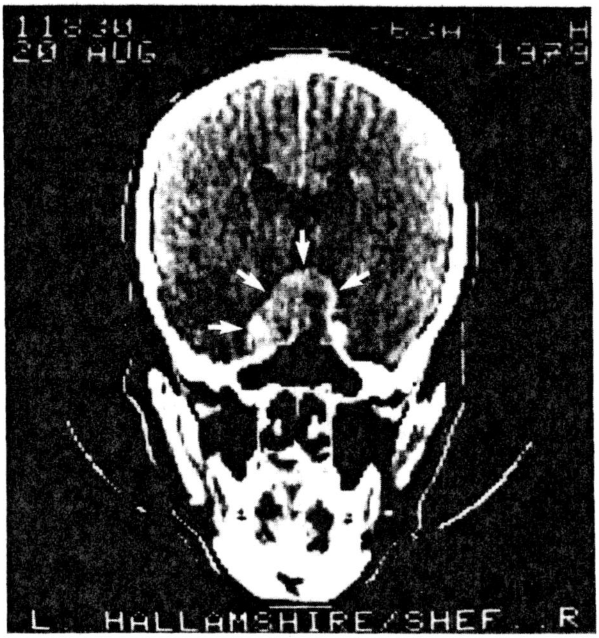

Figure 42a. CT brain scan (enhanced) showing pituitary adenoma (recurrent).

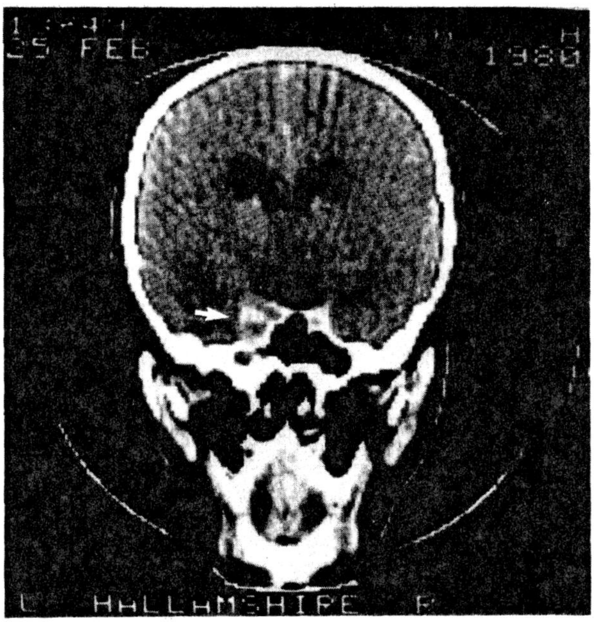

Figure 42b. Six months later: small residual parasellar mass after radiotherapy.

15. Opportunistic infection

Patients suffering from malignant disease show an increased susceptibility to infection. This susceptibility may be manifested not only by ordinary infection but by the occurrence of protozoal, viral and fungal diseases which in the general population are extremely rare. Such infections are termed opportunistic. There are three main reasons for the occurrence of such infections. Firstly, there may be a depression of immunological competence associated with the malignant process. Secondly, cytotoxic chemotherapy and the use of corticosteroid drugs often have an adverse effect on the operation of immunological mechanisms. Thirdly, the need to treat ordinary infections with broad spectrum antibodies may predispose to the unusual diseases mentioned above.

One of the commonest infections is candidiasis of the oesophagus. While this is undoubtedly a distressing and painful condition for the patient, recognition by clinical and radiological means is usually straight-forward and in no way does the presentation mimic the recurrence of malignant disease. Accordingly, in the context of the assessment of response to treatment the appearance of oesophageal candidiasis does not cloud the issue.

In contrast the occurrence of opportunistic infection in the lung may cause shadows to appear on the chest radiograph which may mimic the recurrence of malignancy. It is important, therefore, to be aware of the possibility of such infections and of the radiological patterns which they may cause. Organisms causing opportunistic infection include the following:

1) Pneumocystis carinii;
2) Candida albicans;
3) Aspergillus fumigatus;
4) Cryptococcus neoformans;
5) Nocardia asteroides.

In addition to the above organisms which are otherwise uncommon invaders of the lung, it should be remembered that the commoner organisms including the tubercle bacillus, staphylococci, pneumococci and gram negative organisms may also cause lung infections of unusually florid nature.

15.1. Pneumocystis carinii pneumonia

It is of particular importance to recognize the radiological pattern caused by this organism which in conjunction with the clinical presentation enables the diagnosis of an essentially treatable disease to be made [40]. Clinically a

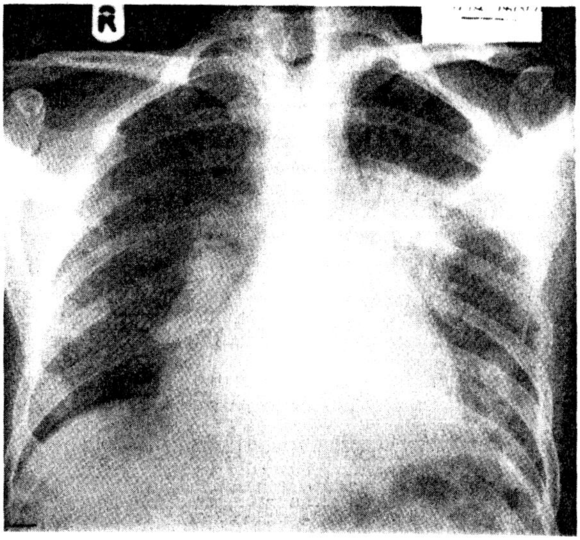

Figure 43. Pneumocystis carinii pneumonia.

patient, most commonly suffering from one of the lymphomas and having been treated with multi-agent chemotherapy, presents with a low-grade fever, shortness of breath and evidence of an alveolar-capillary block. The chest radiograph (Fig. 43) shows a dense bilateral peri-hilar infiltrate densely confluent in the immediate peri-hilar region and becoming less dense and more granular in pattern in its more peripheral parts. The alveolar nature of the process is illustrated by the accompanying air bronchogram pattern. There is evidence of reduced lung compliance in that the diaphragms do not descend to the usual extent on full inspiration. The infecting organism is protozoal in nature and its life cycle is largely unknown. Its presence as an infecting organism may be recognized in suitable stained lung tissue where characteristic cysts may be found. Less commonly those cysts are also seen in the sputum. The diagnosis may be made by lung biopsy best carried out by the transbronchial technique. The older open biopsy is no longer necessary but the percutaneous needle technique may yield satisfactory material.

The importance of establishing the diagnosis lies in the treatability of the infection using co-trimoxazole in high doses. Alternatively pentamidine may be used but is more toxic.

A high proportion of patients with lymphoma showing the above presentation and radiological appearances will have Pneumocystis carinii pneumonia [41]. Less typical cases, however, may resemble the radiological appearances of cryptococcal and aspergillus infections.

15.2. Candida albicans pneumonia

The appearances in this infection are much less specific. Multiple areas of ill-defined pulmonary shadowing, mainly of a linear nature, are seen in the mid and lower zones of the lung fields. The radiological appearances are non-specific but the concurrence of candidal oesophagitis may indicate the probable infecting organism in the lung.

15.3. Aspergillus fumigatus

Lung infections due to this organism have a wider variety of radiological appearances including bilateral diffuse pneumonia, multiple lung opacities which may or may not cavitate, a solitary well-defined mass which again may cavitate and multiple thin-walled cavities complicating a previous patchy consolidation (possibly tension pneumatocoeles of a similar nature to those seen in staphylococcal pneumonia). It is not usually possible to make a specific diagnosis of aspergillus infection on the basis of a chest radiograph and evidence may have to be obtained from the sputum or by serological examination.

It may in some circumstances be very difficult to distinguish between tumour nodules in the chest and infection due to Aspergillus fumigatus.

15.4. Cryptococcus neoformans

Cryptococcal pneumonia is of a non-specific bronchopneumonic pattern showing no characteristic radiological features. It is difficult to treat despite the availability of therapeutic agents active against the organism and is often a terminal event (Fig. 44).

15.5. Nocardia asteroides

Infection with the fungal organism Nocardia produces multiple rounded pulmonary opacities which rapidly cavitate [42]. The appearances may mimic recurrent tumour nodules in the chest.

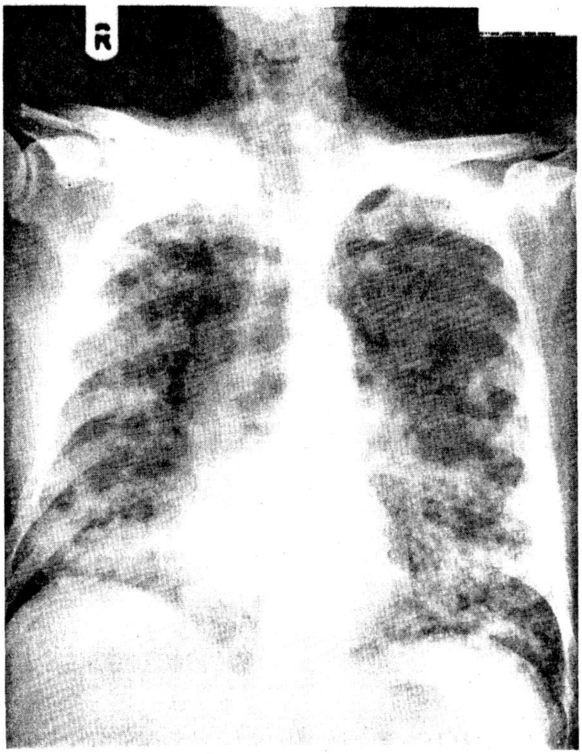

Figure 44. Cryptococcus neoformans pneumonia.

16. Lung abnormalities due to the effects of radiation and certain drugs

Shadows mimicking malignant pulmonary infiltrates may occur both as a response to radiation therapy to the lung and following the use of certain chemotherapeutic agents.

Radiation damage to the lung appears initially at about six to ten weeks after the completion of radiotherapy. At this time linear or confluent shadows appear in the area of the radiation field and are slowly replaced by more clearly defined linear densities due to fibrosis. Accompanying shrinkage of the lung tissue may be noted distorting the outline of the previously identifiable radiation field. The development of the changes may not be fully complete until eighteen months after the radiation therapy.

Confusion with recurrent malignancy is unlikely to occur except in the early stages of a confluent pulmonary shadow. At this time the relationship to the recent radiotherapy should clarify the diagnosis.

A large number of drugs is now known to cause diffuse lung disease. Many of these are not relevant in the context of the differential diagnosis of lung opacities in patients with malignant disease. However, diffuse interstitial (reticulonodular) lung infiltration may be produced by busulfan, Bleomycin, methotrexate, cyclophosphamide and BCNU. Clearly the potential resemblance of these appearances to lymphangitis carcinomatosa may cause a diagnostic difficulty to occur. It should also be noted that the occurrence of such drug reactions is often associated with fever, thus causing the presentation to resemble that of an opportunistic lung infection. In this situation a lung biopsy may be the only means of establishing the diagnosis [43]. It may be important to establish a definite diagnosis since the lung changes associated with the above chemotherapeutic drugs may in some circumstances be reversible though in the case of busulfan induced lung disease some permanent lung damage is usually a feature.

References

1. Husband JE, Peckham MJ, MacDonald JS, Hendry WF: The role of computed tomography in the management of testicular teratoma. Clin Radiol 30:243–252, 1979.
2. King DJ, Dawson AA, McDonald AF: Gallium scanning in lymphoma. Clin Radiol 31:729–732, 1980.
3. Kreel L: Computerized tomography using the EMI general purpose scanner. Br J Radiol 50:2–14, 1977.
4. Kinmonth JB, Kemp-Harper RA, Taylor GW: Lymphangiography by radiological methods. J Fac Radiol 6:217–223, 1955.
5. MacDonald JS, Peckham MJ: Lymphography in Hodgkin's disease, pp 169–178. In: Hodgkin's disease, Smithers DW (ed). Edinburgh: Churchill Livingstone, 1973.
6. Glees JP, Gazet JC, MacDonald JS, Peckham MJ: The accuracy of lymphography in Hodgkin's disease. Clin Radiol 25:5–11, 1974.
7. Castellino RA, Billingham J, Dorfman EF: Lymphographic accuracy in Hodgkin's disease and malignant lymphoma with a note on the 'reactive' lymph node as a cause of most false positive lymphograms. Invest Radiol 9:155–165, 1974.
8. Wilkinson DJ, MacDonald JS: A review of the role of lymphography in the management of testicular tumours. Clin Radiol 26:155–165, 1974.
9. Wallace S, Jing BS: Lymphangiography: diagnosis of nodal metastases from testicular malignancies. JAMA 213:94–96, 1970.
10. Piver MS, Wallace S, Castro JR: The accuracy of lymphangiography in carcinoma of the uterine cervix. Am J Roentgenol 111:278–283, 1971.
11. Lecart C, Lenfant P: Critical appraisal of lymphangiography in cancer of the female genital tract. Lymphology 4:100–108, 1971.
12. Vinje B, Skjennald A, Fryjordet A: Lymphography in the evaluation of urinary bladder carcinoma. Clin Radiol 31:551–553, 1980.
13. Turner AG, Hendry WF, MacDonald JS, Wallace DM: The value of lymphography in the management of bladder cancer. Br J Urol 48:579–586, 1976.

14. Rodger A, Wild SR, Duncan W: Bipedal lymphography in the management of bladder cancer. Clin Radiol 31:555–558, 1980.
15. Williams MV, MacDonald JS, Peckham MJ: Changes in the size of pelvic lymph nodes in patients being followed after radiotherapy for Hodgkin's disease. Clin Radiol 31:545–550, 1980.
16. Carr D, Davidson JK: Magnification lymphography. Clin Radiol 31:535–539, 1980.
17. Kaplan HS, Dorfman RF, Nelson TS, Rosenberg SA: Staging laparotomy and splenectomy in Hodgkin's disease: analysis of the indications and patterns of involvement in 285 consecutive patients. National Cancer Institute Monograph, 36, 291, 1973.
18. Kadin ME, Glatstein E, Dorfman RF: Clinicopathological studies of 117 untreated patients subjected to laparotomy for the staging of Hodgkin's disease. Cancer 27:1277–1294, 1971.
19. National Lymphoma Group Report. The value of laparotomy and splenectomy in the management of early Hodgkin's disease. Clin Radiol 26:151–157, 1975.
20. Crowther D, Blackledge G, Best JK: The role of computed tomography of the abdomen in the diagnosis and staging of patients with lymphoma. Clin Haematol 8(3):567–591, 1979.
21. Lee JKT, McClennan BL, Stanley RJ, Sagel SS: Computed tomography in the staging of testicular neoplasms. Radiology 130:387–390, 1979.
22. Meire HB: Diagnostic ultrasound. Br J Radiol 52:685–703, 1979.
23. Filly RA, Marglin S, Castellino RA: The ultrasonographic spectrum of abdominal and pelvic Hodgkin's disease and non-Hodgkin's lymphoma. Cancer 38:2143–2148, 1976.
24. Ennis MG, MacErlean DP: Percutaneous aspiration biopsy of abdomen and retroperitoneum. Clin Radiol 31:611–616, 1980.
25. Requard CK, Mettler FA: The use of ultrasound in the evaluation of trophoblastic disease and in its response to therapy. Radiology 135:419–422, 1980.
26. Photopulos GJ, McCartney WH, Walton LA, Staab EV: Computerized tomography applied to gynecologic oncology. Am J Obstet Gynecol 135:381–383, 1979.
27. Amendola MA, Walsh JW, Amendola BE, Tisnado J, Hall DJ, Goplerud DR: Computed tomography in the evaluation of carcinoma of the ovary. J Comput Assist Tomogr 5:179–186, 1981.
28. Brooke JR, Palubinskas AJ, Federle MP: CT evaluation of invasive lesions of the bladder. J Comput Assist Tomogr 5:22–26, 1981.
29. Ding-Jen L, Leibel S, Shiels R, Sanders R, Siegelman S, Order S: The value of ultrasonic imaging and CT scanning in planning the radiotherapy for prostatic carcinoma. Cancer 45:724–727, 1980.
30. Segal RL, Zuckerman H, Friedman EW: Soft tissue roentgenography. Its use in diagnosis of thyroid carcinoma. J Am Med Assoc 173:1890–1894, 1960.
31. MacDonald JS: The diagnosis of tumours of the thyroid, p 196. In: Tumours of the thyroid gland, Smithers D (ed). Edinburgh: E. & S. Livingstone, 1970.
32. Merrick MV: Bone scanning. Br J Radiol 48:327–351, 1975.
33. Castronovo FP, Callaghan RJ, Potsaid MS, Pendergrass HP: Effects of radiation therapy on bone lesions as measured by 99Tcm-diphosphonate. J Nucl Med 14:604–605, 1973.
34. McNeil BJ, Cassady JR, Geisler CF, Jaffe N, Traggis D, Treves S: Fluorine 18 bone scintigraphy in children with osteosarcoma or Ewing's sarcoma: Radiology 109:627–631, 1973.
35. Edelstyn GA, Gillespie PJ, Grebell FS: The radiological demonstration of osseous metastases. Clin Radiol 18:158–162, 1967.
36. Gynning I, Langeland P, Lindberg S, Waldeskog B: Localisation with Sr 85 of spinal metastases in mammary cancer and changes in uptake after hormone and roentgen therapy. Acta Radiol (Diagn) (Stockh) 55:119–128, 1961.

37. Harbert JC, Ashburn WL: Radiostrontium bone scanning in Hodgkin's disease. Cancer 22:58–63, 1968.
38. Parsons CA, Chapman P, Counter RT, Grundy A: The role of computed tomography in tumours of the larynx. Clin Radiol 31:529–533, 1980.
39. Taylor KJW: Ultrasound scanning of the spleen, p 170. In: Atlas of grey scale ultrasonography, Taylor KJW (ed). New York: Churchill-Livingstone, 1978.
40. Western KA, Perera DR, Schultz MG: Pentamidine isethionate in the treatment of pneumocystis carinii pneumonia. Ann Intern Med 73:695–702, 1970.
41. Goodell B, Jacobs JB, Powell RD, De Vita VT: Pneumocystis carinii: the spectrum of diffuse interstitial pneumonia in patients with neoplastic diseases. Ann Intern Med 172:337–340, 1970.
42. Hatfield PM: Cavitating pulmonary nodules complicating Hodgkin's disease. J Am Med Assoc 215:1145–1146, 1971.
43. Greenman RL, Goodall PT, King D: Lung biopsy in immunocompromised hosts. Am J Med 59:488–496, 1975.
44. Morrison DA, Goldman AL: Radiographic patterns of drug-induced lung disease. Radiology 131:299–304, 1979.

3. Tumour Markers

A. MILFORD WARD

1. Introduction

Tumour markers may be defined as serum or body fluid constituents found in inappropriate concentrations in tumour bearing patients. As such they encompass not only those products of tumour cells which may correctly be termed tumour antigens but also normal body constituents that are produced in excessive amounts in response to the tumour load. Tumour antigens are 'synthetic' markers and these may be tumour specific like the oncofetal antigens or nonspecific like the various enzyme and hormones that may demonstrate inappropriate secretion. Those substances produced by host tissues as a response to the presence of tumour are 'reactive' markers and include such substances as the acute phase reactive proteins and many enzymes. These reactive markers can never be considered as specific for the tumour bearing state and their interpretation should always be approached with caution.

Table 1. Tumour markers

SYNTHETIC	Tumour specific	Oncofetal antigens/proteins Proteins
	Non-specific	Proteins Hormones Enzymes Nucleosides
REACTIVE	Non-specific	Acute phase proteins Enzymes

With few notable exceptions, the specificity of tumour markers for any particular malignancy is poor and, indeed, many of the synthetic markers may, on occasion, be considered as acute phase reactive substances, found as they are in increased concentrations in some inflammatory diseases. These synthetic markers with acute phase properties are, for the most part, cell surface antigens which are liberated during situations of increased cell turnover which may occur in regenerative states as well as in malignancy.

Tumour markers are conventionally thought of as recent innovations dependent on modern technology for their characterisation and measure-

Hancock, B. W. (ed.), Assessment of Tumour Response.
 ISBN 90-247-2712-X.
Printed in The Netherlands.

ment. It is salutary, therefore, to remember that the most specific and sensitive marker in the armamentarium of the laboratory was first described in 1847. Bence Jones [1] characterised the protein by which he is eponymically remembered but which had been previously isolated by MacIntyre [2] from the patient described by Dalrymple [3]. Bence Jones Protein or, more correctly, monoclonal free immunoglobulin light chains, in the urine is specific for plasma cell malignancy and is virtually never seen in any other situation. Such specificity cannot be claimed for any other tumour marker in general use today.

Despite the veritable plethora of tumour markers described in the last two decades relatively few have stood the test of time and been shown to be of clinical value. The major question that must be asked of all putative markers is, 'does the marker level allow the clinician to plan patient management?'. The answer to this question is at best a qualified 'yes' in a small group of marker substances and then only in the light of the established clinical status.

1.1. Alpha fetoprotein (AFP)

AFP is a normal serum protein of the fetus first described by Bergstrand and Czar [4]. It is a glycoprotein of 65 000 dalton with a biological half-life of 3.5–4.0 days. It is synthesised in the fetal liver, foregut and yolk sac from the 10th gestational week [5]. Molecular heterogeneity based on the structure of the carbohydrate moeity has been described [6] which allows distinction to be made between AFP of hepatic and yolk sac origin.

The role of AFP as a tumour marker was first claimed by Abelev [7] by his description of elevated levels in the serum of mice with transplantable hepatocellular carcinomas. This was closely followed by Tatarinov's description of elevated levels in human hepatocellular carcinoma [8] and somewhat later by the description of similar elevations in certain germ cell tumours [9]. The origin of the gonadal tumour AFP in yolk sac elements [10] of the teratomatous tumours successfully linked the physiological state described by Gitlin with the pathological morphology of Teilum [11].

1.2. Human chorionic gonadotrophin (HCG)

HCG is a placental glycoprotein hormone of 38 000 dalton with a biological half-life of rather less than 24 h. It is synthesised by the syncytial trophoblast and by non-gestational trophoblast elements in both gonadal and extra gonadal tumours. HCG is composed of two dissimilar polypeptide chains.

The α chain is identical to the α chains of human luteinising hormone (LH) and follicle stimulating hormone (FSH). The β chain, whilst being distinct from that of FSH, shares 86 identical residues with the β chain of LH differing only in the extra C terminal domain of 26 residues. Whilst total HCG is used as a marker for intrauterine choriocarcinoma, tumour specificity for extrauterine malignancy is achieved by assay of the β subunit. In addition to its secretion by trophoblastic elements in germ cell tumours, inappropriate secretion has been described in a wide variety of malignancies [12].

The lack of total specificity of most antisera for the β subunit of HCG leads to varying degrees of cross reactivity with endogenous LH and spurious elevations of the marker, particularly in female patients. LH is also known to rise after orchidectomy. This, together with the rise associated with chemotherapy-induced hypogonadism, will explain some of the spurious elevations noted in males undergoing regular βHCG monitoring of gonadal tumour therapy. Reassay after administration of testosterone may resolve any diagnostic problems that may arise [13].

1.3. Carcinoembryonic antigen (CEA)

Carcinoembryonic antigen is a family of acid glycoproteins of about 200 000 dalton which demonstrate considerable intermolecular and intramolecular heterogeneity. Originally it was described as carcinoembryonic antigen (CEA) of the human digestive system to denote its site of isolation and preparation. It is expressed in considerable amounts by the fetal intestinal epithelium where it can be found in the glycocalyx surrounding the cell membrane and from whence it can be shed into the circulation [14]. CEA can be detected as a normal serum protein in the adult at concentrations of less than 2.5 μg/l. Modest elevations may be found during pregnancy in smokers and in certain inflammatory diseases such as ulcerative colitis, Crohn's disease and pulmonary infections. Raised levels may also be seen in association with some benign tumours. Grossly raised levels, in excess of 20 μg/l, are, however, strongly suggestive of malignancy.

As a tumour marker it suffers from low sensitivity (true positive rate) and poor specificity (true negative rate), and cannot, therefore, be used reliably as diagnostic agent for population screening or in the 'at risk' patient. Its value as a monitor of tumour elimination is hampered by a failure to define an acceptable biological half-life, estimates ranging from 6 to 60 days being reported [15]. This gross variation in biological half-life estimates is related to the molecular heterogeneity and to the more rapid elimination of deglycosylated components.

Regular and sequential assay of CEA does, however, have a role in the management of colorectal, breast and bronchial carcinoma.

1.4. Oncofetal pancreatic antigen (OPA)

Oncofetal Pancreatic Antigen (OPA) [16, 17] is one of a group of oncofetal antigens described in relation to carcinoma of pancreas. OPA is described as having a molecular weight of about 40 000 dalton and to be relatively low in carbohydrate. As a marker of carcinoma of pancreas, OPA has good sensitivity but only moderate specificity. Some overlap in assay values is seen in cases of chronic pancreatitis, and OPA synthesis is seen in cases of other foregut derived tumours. The finding of postoperative decline in OPA values following successful resection of pancreatic carcinoma suggests that this antigen may have a place in the management of this notoriously refractory malignancy.

1.5. Pregnancy specific β glycoprotein (SP1)

Pregnancy Specific β Glycoprotein (SPl) is a glycoprotein of trophoblastic origin which has been examined as a potential second marker for choriocarcinoma and the trophoblastic elements of gonadal teratomas. The few cases where there is discordance between SPl and HCG in relation to trophoblastic tumour load suggests that there may be differing responses to therapy within the metabolic pathways of the two markers [18]. The differences are, however, not sufficient to justify the inclusion of SP1 in the monitoring schedule at the present time.

1.6. Monoclonal immunoglobulins (MIg) and immunoglobulin fragments

Neoplastic proliferation of a single clone of immunoglobulin producing cells leads to the production of a quantity of identical molecules which migrate on electrophoresis of serum or urine as a discrete abnormal band. This abnormal protein component has been variously termed 'paraprotein', 'M-component', or 'monoclonal component'. It is a true synthetic tumour marker in that it is the product of a neoplastic secretory cell line. Unbalanced immunoglobulin chain production by the neoplastic cell leads to an excess of free light chains which may appear in the urine where they demonstrate the unique thermo-solubility characteristics which has earned them the eponymic name of Bence Jones Protein.

The neoplastic plasma cell proliferation is also associated with a reduction or paresis of the non-neoplastic immunoglobulin producing cell lines. The protein abnormality required as one of the diagnostic criteria of myelomatosis [19] includes the presence of a serum or urine monoclonal component or an immune paresis.

Differentiation of the neoplastic from the benign monoclonal gammopathy is made by the relentless progression and increase in concentration of the neoplastic monoclonal component and the presence of the excess monoclonal free light chains. Monoclonal components may be seen as an age related phenomenon with an increasing frequency after the age of 60 years [20]. Whilst many of these are benign, a proportion do have malignant potential [21].

1.7. Prostatic acid phosphatase (PAP)

The tartrate labile isoenzyme of acid phosphatase has long been used as a diagnostic test for carcinoma of the prostate [22]. Despite the long years of use PAP is neither a sensitive nor a specific marker for carcinoma of prostate in its early stages. The advent of a specific radioimmunoassay [23] has done little to increase the sensitivity of the assay but has helped considerably in the specificity. Whilst with the enzymatic technique 50–70% of bony metastases [24] from carcinoma of prostate give elevated values, this proportion can be increased to better than 90% by the immunoassay [23].

1.8. Acute phase reactant proteins (APRP)

The acute phase reactant proteins, α_1 acidglycoprotein, haptoglobin, ceruloplasmin, α_1 antitrypsin, and α_1 antichymotrypsin, are all known to rise in tumour bearing patients [25]. The response is reactive on the part of the host and entirely nonspecific. Similar profile changes may also be seen in inflammatory and degenerative conditions and can never be taken as diagnostic of malignancy. They do, however, offer some small advantage in the long-term monitoring of patients treated for established malignant disease.

A linear discriminant function analysis involving concurrent assay of a profile of APRPs and CEA has been shown to have prognostic significance in relation to carcinoma of the colon [26]. Sequential analyses in the postoperative period could also demonstrate recurrence better than with CEA alone but this system suffers from the stimulating effect of trauma on APRP synthesis, making many of the values totally unreliable in the first month after surgery.

A similar approach can be taken with carcinoma of prostate with the substitution of prostatic acid phosphatase as the specific marker in place of

CEA [27]. This discriminant can satisfactorily identify extracapsular spread of the tumour with a greater sensitivity and accuracy than bone scanning and at less trauma to the patient than pelvic node biopsy. The value of local metastasis identification in patient management is, however, doubtful. Te Velde *et al.* [28] have shown a similar value of acute phase reactant proteins in identifying recurrence in patients with carcinoma of cervix. These workers claim a 3–4 month lead time on the basis of serial estimations of α_1 antitrypsin, Cl esterase inhibitor and C reactive protein.

Bradwell [29] showed a significant relationship between haptoglobin and α_1 acid glycoprotein levels and tumour mass in carcinoma of bronchus. There was also a significant relationship between α_1 acid glycoprotein concentrations and survival. This relationship was independent of the original concentration and tumour mass and may reflect silent metastatic disease at the time of primary surgery. Both haptoglobin and α_1 acid glycoprotein were shown to rise on average 4 months before the clinical appearance of metastatic disease and with a greater reliability than CEA. The picture was, however, confused by the acute phase response to any episode of pulmonary infection to which such patients are particularly prone.

Other reports have shown a close stage relationship between carcinoma of the bladder [30], carcinoma of the cervix [31] and non-Hodgkins lymphoma [32] and the acute phase reactant profile. Whilst this relationship cannot be considered diagnostic, it can be of value in the pretreatment assessment of the therapeutic options.

2. Tumour markers and primary diagnosis

The specificity of even the synthetic markers is in general too low to allow their reliable use as primary diagnostic aids. Although the initial studies with carcinoembryonic antigen (CEA) [33] suggested it to be both a sensitive and specific marker for adenocarcinoma of the colon, further studies have shown it to be produced by many tumour types and to be present in increased concentrations in a number of inflammatory or reactive states. There is now general agreement that only 40% of Stage I adenocarcinoma of the colon are CEA positive and that any attempted screening programme would be faced with a similar 40% false positive rate. A similar situation can be found with most other tumour markers.

The relatively few markers that can be considered of proven value in primary diagnosis are listed in Table 2 and even here due consideration must be given to the clinical situation in which the assay is attempted. Alpha fetoprotein (AFP) can only be considered as a diagnostic marker in the situation of a possible hepatic tumour in the very young child. Human

Table 2. Tumour markers of value in primary diagnosis

1. Alphafetoprotein	Hepatoblastoma
2. Bence Jones protein	Plasmacytoma and myeloma
3. HCG	Choriocarcinoma

chorionic gonadatrophin (HCG) is similarly of diagnostic significance only in a woman who has previously had a hydatidiform mole and is known not to be pregnant.

Table 3 includes some of the more recently described markers which have no value in primary diagnosis, their specificity or sensitivity being such that the false negative and false positive results will significantly exceed the number of correct diagnoses made.

Table 3. Tumour markers unreliable in primary diagnosis

Carcinoembryonic antigen (CEA)
Casein
Fetal sulphaglycoprotein antigen (FSA)
Isoferritin (α_2H)
Non-cross-reacting antigen (NCA)
Pregnancy associated macroglobulin (PAM, SP3)
Tenessee antigen
Tissue polypeptide antigen (TPA)

There is, however, a third group in which, under specific clinical circumstances, the presence of tumour markers may give a useful guide or indication to the primary diagnosis. Some of these are detailed in Table 4. AFP, βHCG and SPl can all present guides to the diagnosis in a patient with a gonadal mass and, by virtue of their cytological origin, can give a guide to the histological appearance of the tumour and its prognosis.

Table 4. Tumour markers of value as a guide to diagnosis

1. Alphafeto protein.	Gonadal teratoma (yolk sac elements).
2. Carcinoembryonic antigen in pancreatic juice.	Carcinoma of pancreas.
3. Oncofetal pancreatic antigen.	Carcinoma of pancreas.
4. Thyrocalcitonin.	Medullary carcinoma of thyroid.
5. Pregnancy specific β glycoprotein (SP1).	Gonadal teratoma (trophoblastic elements).
6. β subunit human chorionic gonadotrophin.	Gonadal teratoma (trophoblastic elements).
7. Excessive levels of many markers.	

Oncofetal pancreatic antigen (OPA), whilst being found in many tumours of the foregut derivatives, may be of considerable value in the differential diagnosis of an obstructive jaundice as will also the CEA level in pancreatic juice.

Gross excess of any marker may be considered diagnostic of the tumour bearing state, but site of origin remains a clinical decision, although this may be considered as rather academic when the excessive marker levels are usually associated with Stage IV disease.

2.1. AFP in hepatoblastoma and hepatocellular carcinoma

AFP elevations above 50–100 μg/l are seen in all cases of hepatoblastoma of childhood and in 80–90% of hepatocellular carcinoma in adults [34, 35, 36]. Sustained elevations of AFP can vary enormously in magnitude from the modest elevations of 100 μg/l to several g/l [37].

The demonstration of AFP elevations prior to the development of liver tumours in genetically predisposed animals [38] and following ingestion of hepatic carcinogens [39] have raised the possibility of using AFP as a screening test for hepatocellular carcinoma in man. The temporal relationship between onset of hepatic malignancy and the elevation of measurable levels of AFP in man is unclear. The situation is further confused by possible racial differences in reference values and the effect of endemic hepatitis, hepatic regeneration following hepatitis being associated with temporary elevations of AFP [40]. The incidence of hepatocellular carcinoma in Europe and the U.S. is too low to warrant population screening except in selected populations where there is a recognised carcinogenic risk [41]. Repetitive testing in this situation is essential as only sustained and increasing levels may be considered as indicative of malignancy.

One mass screening programme is recorded [42] where 500 000 individuals were screened for the possible development of hepatocellular carcinoma. Several were detected and 10% showed a biphasic response on serial studies similar to that seen in chemical carcinogenesis [39].

2.2. AFP in other abdominal malignancy

In keeping with the synthesis of AFP by the fetal foregut, there are occasional reports of AFP elevations in association with tumours arising from foregut derivatives. Rare AFP producing tumours of the stomach, duodenum and pancreas have been described [43]. This situation is more likely to introduce confusion into the diagnosis rather than be of assistance, on account of the rarity of the situation.

3. Tumour markers in the monitoring of malignancy

The logical and appropriate use of tumour markers is in the field of monitoring of therapy and the early detection of recurrent disease. In this role tumour markers have a valuable part to play in the modern management of malignant disease.

Table 5. The role of tumour markers in the monitoring of malignant disease

1. Indicators of residual tumours
   a) for second look surgery
   b) selection for adjuvant therapy
2. Early diagnosis of recurrent disease
   a) lead time for therapy
   b) early assessment of clinical trials
3. Response to therapy
   a) assessment of the effect of adjuvant therapy
   b) indication for change of therapy

The three main lines of approach in relation to the use of tumour markers in the monitoring of malignant disease are listed in Table 5. The serum level of the synthetic markers is related to the tumour load within fairly broad confines. In the teratoma group the AFP and βHCG levels will relate to the mass of yolk sac or trophoblastic tissue, respectively, rather than to the total tumour bulk. In the plasma cell malignancies the relationship of monoclonal component concentration to tumour bulk in different patients is much less marked unless the subclass of the monoclonal immunoglobulin is defined. Even with this proviso the relationship is weak and estimates of tumour load are more reliably restricted to relative assessment within the one patient.

The rate of elimination of a marker after primary, or successful adjuvant, therapy is a complex calculation involving the doubling time of the tumour, the marker synthetic rate and its biological half-life or catabolic rate.

Marker kinetics, where they can be calculated, offer an earlier indication of successful therapy than can be obtained by awaiting basal levels which may never be achieved. This has been applied most satisfactorily to the decay of AFP levels following orchidectomy for testicular teratoma. The Apparent Half Life (AHL) after treatment should approximate the biological half-life of the protein if there has been complete elimination of marker producing tissue [44]. The slope of the marker regression curve derived from sequential sample analysis can be expressed as

$$\mathrm{AHL} = \frac{-0.693\,\mathrm{T}}{\log_e \dfrac{(\mathrm{Ct})}{(\mathrm{Co})}}$$

where T is the interval in days between marker analyses, Ct is the concentration at time T and Co the initial marker concentration. For AFP, with a biological half-life of 3.5–4.0 days, values for the AHL in excess of 5 days are indicative of residual disease which will eventually recur, whilst values in excess of 10 days carry an extremely bad prognosis with large volume residual disease and the probability of early recurrence. AHL values of less than 5 days are invariably associated with Stage I disease and carry an excellent prognosis. This is essentially similar to, but rather simpler than, the Lange [45] approach where the expected AFP concentration X_t is compared with the observed level in the patient.

$$X_t = X_0 \, e^{-0.139\,t}$$

(X_0 is the initial concentration and X_t the concentration after t days). Although most studies using this approach have concentrated on marker decay following primary surgical treatment it can also be used following adjuvant therapy aimed at elimination of residual tumour load.

The marker kinetics or rate of postoperative elimination of a marker are sensitive indicators of residual disease.

Marker recurrence after an initial fall may be indicative of the need for second look surgery to remove residual disease, whilst a prolonged AHL indicates the need for adjuvant therapy. Sequential monitoring over many weeks or months allows the early diagnosis of recurrent disease and may give a lead time of up to six months on the development of clinical symptoms. Marker recurrence as opposed to clinical recurrence can also give an earlier indication of the effectiveness of a therapeutic regimen and allow earlier assessment of clinical trials of new chemotherapeutic agents.

This response to therapy can also be used to indicate the need to change a patient from one agent to another if marker elimination is not being achieved. Early assessment of the effectiveness or otherwise of a therapeutic regimen may considerably affect the eventual outcome in the individual patient and obviate the unnecessary use of toxic agents to no effect.

4. The use of tumour markers in the management of specific malignancies

4.1. Choriocarcinoma

Serum levels of βHCG are measured routinely after uterine evacuation in all cases of hydatidiform mole and as a monitor of chemotherapy in choriocarcinoma [46]. In these situations βHCG is an ideal marker, albeit of a relatively rare tumour. It can be used to good clinical effect both to monitor therapy and to diagnose recurrent disease. As the 'at-risk' population is small and definable, it is also logistically possible to use the marker as a screening test for the development of the malignancy. The serum levels correlate closely with tumour load and increased levels may be detected with a minimum of 10^5 cells [47].

Central nervous system involvement may be accurately predicted by estimation of βHCG levels in the CSF [48].

4.2. Germ cell tumours

Ninety percent of all testicular teratomas show elevations of either AFP or βHCG; in many instances both markers are elevated [49, 50]. Similar elevations of either or both markers may be seen in malignant teratoma of ovary and extragonadal sites. βHCG elevations are also seen in a proportion of cases of seminoma usually associated with the presence of syncytial giant cells [51].

The combined use of both markers is crucial to the adequate management of germ cell tumours in all sites, both gonadal [52, 53] and extragonadal [54].

4.2.1. Staging. Elevated levels of either marker prior to surgical excision will fall to normal in Stage I disease within the biological half-life of the marker [44, 50, 55]. Falling marker levels and AHL estimates can only be observed if regular serum samples are taken for assay. Table 6 gives details of the recommended schedule for adequate monitoring of all germ cell tumours by regular assay of AFP and βHCG.

Table 6. Protocol for marker monitoring of germ cell tumour therapy

1. Serum for AFP and βHCG on first examination.
2. Repeat serum prior to operation or primary treatment.
3. Repeat serum twice weekly after primary treatment: continue for eight weeks or until marker levels become basal.
4. Weekly samples for six months: if no clinical or marker recurrence
5. Monthly samples: in the absence of clinical or marker recurrence, monitoring can cease after 3 years.

In testicular teratoma marker decay with an AHL for AFP of greater than 5 days indicates residual disease, and the possible need for retroperitoneal lymph node dissection. Elevated marker levels on follow-up without positive clinical or investigational findings are considered as minimal bulk metastatic disease (Stage IIs) [56] and are of guarded prognosis. Rising levels after primary surgery indicate massive residual disease and the overall prognosis is bleak. Whilst much of the available data refers to experiences with testicular germ tumours, the pattern of progression and prognosis is similar for germ cell tumours of ovarian and extragonadal origin [55, 57].

4.2.2. Prognosis. Marker levels are a useful indicator of tumour load prior to surgery and can give a reliable prognostic indication for testicular teratoma. βHCG levels greater than 1×10^5 IU/litre and AFP greater than 1×10^3 IU/litre are associated with a 40% one year mortality [58, 59]. In contrast, βHCG less than 5×10^4 IU/litre or AFP less than 0.5×10^3 IU/litre is only associated with a 10% mortality. Similar prognostic value can be gained from the AHL data where, for AFP in endodermal sinus tumours, an AHL of less than 5 days has an excellent prognosis; for an AHL of 5–10 days the prognosis is guarded with 75% recurrence inside two years; where the AHL exceeds 10 days the one year mortality rate is almost total [55, 57]. There is evidence to suggest that marker levels give a better prognostic index than can be achieved by assessment of tumour bulk [60].

4.2.3. Monitoring therapy. With current curative therapeutic regimes [52, 61, 62], it is imperative that adequate therapy is given. The assessment of adequate therapy is largely gauged by the serial monitor of marker levels for many months after the initial treatment (Table 6). It has been suggested that therapy should continue for 12 weeks after marker levels have become basal [59] or for a total of six courses of combination therapy after that basal point is reached [57]; further maintenance therapy would seem to offer no benefit. Marker monitoring should continue on a monthly basis for at least two years after therapy has been discontinued.

It should be remembered that AFP and βHCG are markers of specific cell types within the germ cell tumour. Advancing clinical disease in the absence of marker elevations indicates selection of non marker producing elements and calls for a change in the therapeutic regimen. In this situation a non specific marker such as ferritin may be of value [63].

4.3. Colorectal carcinoma

Despite much work on the value of CEA in the diagnosis and monitoring of this group of malignancies, the picture remains unclear [64].

4.3.1. Staging. Elevated serum CEA levels are only seen in 20–30% of Stage I or Dukes A tumours compared with 75–80% of patients with hepatic metastases. Site of the tumour within the colorectal axis may also have an effect on CEA production, higher levels being seen in cases of left colonic and sigmoid tumours, whilst lower levels are seen in right colonic and rectal tumours [65].

4.3.2. Prognosis. Gross elevations usually indicate widespread disease with hepatic metastases and have a poor prognosis. Little further information can be gained that cannot be gleaned from clinical examination and histological examination of lymph node involvement in the operative specimen. The irregular and relatively low CEA positivity of some early colorectal tumours can be modified by the use of a combined CEA-APRP approach to staging and prognosis assessment.

A linear discriminant analysis utilising CEA, α_1 antitrypsin and α_1 acid glycoprotein [26]

$$I = 6.2 - 2.6(\log_{10} \text{CEA}) - 1.6(\alpha_1\ \text{AT}) + 1.3(\alpha_1\ \text{AGP})$$

allows both preoperative staging and an overall prognostic assessment. I values $> +0.5$ indicate Stage I or Dukes A disease, whilst negative values indicate Stage 3 (Dukes C) or Stage 4 disease. In an initial study 90% of those with a positive value for I showed no recurrence at two years after resection.

4.3.3. Monitoring. The use of CEA as an indicator for second-look surgery has been disappointing. Despite some enthusiastic claims with a clinical lead time of nine months [66], others have been less successful. In addition, a proportion of patients (20–50%) show clinical evidence of recurrent disease without concomitant elevations in CEA [67]. After complete surgical excision the CEA level should fall to normal within six weeks. Failure to observe such a fall in a case with preoperative CEA elevation is strong evidence for residual disease.

Falling CEA levels following chemotherapy or radiotherapy can only be considered suggestive of a positive response, but rising levels are inconsistent with tumour regression and indicate the need to alter the therapeutic regimen.

4.4. Prostatic carcinoma

The assay of the prostatic isoenzyme of acid phosphatase (PAP) has long been used as a diagnostic test for carcinoma of prostate. The advent of the radioimmunoassay for PAP [23] has only marginally increased the specificity and sensitivity of the test over the long established enzymatic method [22]. As a diagnostic marker PAP leaves much to be desired in that the probability of a positive marker elevation being associated with Stage I disease in the symptomless population is less than 1%. In a patient with a palpable prostatic nodule, 30% of Stage I or intracapsular lesions will give a marker elevation. The sensitivity of PAP for extracapsular spread is much improved and, whilst the enzymatic method gave a positivity of

50–75% [24], the immunoassay can improve the identification of distant metastasis to more than 90% [23].

The linking of acute phase proteins to the specific PAP marker can further improve metastasis identification [27]. In the discriminant function

$$I = -0.638 \log_e PAP + 0.767 \log_e PALB - 2.074 \log_e AAT + 0.605 \log_e AGP - 0.911 \log_e HPT + 4.996$$

where PALB, AAT, AGP and HPT in g/l are the serum concentrations of prealbumin, α_1 antitrypsin, acid glycoprotein and haptoglobin respectively, negative values for I indicate extracapsular spread and give better than 90% identification of bone and lymph node metastases. The profile does, however, suffer from the major problem that AAT is subject to genetic variation in concentrations and AAT, AGP and HPT are subject to variation in concentration with oestrogen administration. This latter phenomenon makes the profile unsuitable for use in the patient on standard adjuvant treatment regimens.

Post treatment monitoring with six monthly immunoassay for PAP is an acceptable method of detecting late recurrence and the development of distant metastases.

4.5. Myelomatosis and monoclonal gammopathies

The differentiation between benign and malignant monoclonal gammopathy depends on the former remaining at stable concentrations over at least three years and there being no evidence of associated immune paresis. Where a monoclonal serum component has been identified and bone marrow and radiological examination are normal, the protein abnormality should be monitored by three monthly examination of both serum and urine for at least three years before a firm diagnosis of benign monoclonal gammopathy can be made. Treatment of such an isolated protein abnormality is contra indicated.

The presence of a monoclonal serum or urinary protein abnormality is one of the cornerstones of the diagnosis of myelomatosis [19]. Serial estimates of the paraprotein concentration in serum and of Bence Jones protein in the urine are an excellent guide to tumour mass. Remission can be gauged by the degree or rate of reduction of the monoclonal component. Whilst two or three estimates prior to chemotherapy are useful to indicate growth rate of the tumour, serial estimates on treatment are not necessary more frequently than three monthly unless marked clinical deterioration is noted.

4.5.1. Prognosis. Despite the excellent relationship between monoclonal component and tumour mass, the concentration is not a reliable indicator of prognosis. This is best achieved by attention to the serum albumin concentration [19] or to the haemoglobin and urea levels [68, 69] and to the degree of immune paresis.

Increasing levels of serum paraprotein and/or urinary Bence Jones protein indicate escape from clinical control and require a change in therapeutic management. It should be remembered, however, that some cases of myelomatosis may revert to a more undifferentiated state and lose the ability to synthesise or secrete immunoglobulin. The total disappearance of the monoclonal component should not be taken as evidence of complete remission unless the immune paresis is also reversed.

References

1. Bence Jones H: Papers in chemical pathology. Lancet ii:88–92, 1847.
2. MacIntyre W: Case of mollities and fragilitas ossium. Med Chir Soc Trans 33:211–232, 1846.
3. Dalrymple J: On the microscopic character of mollities ossium. Dublin J Med Sci 2:85–95, 1846.
4. Bergstrand CG, Czar B: Demonstration of a new protein fraction in the serum from a human fetus. Scand J Clin Lab Invest 8:174, 1956.
5. Gitlin D: Normal biology of alphfetoprotein. Ann NY Acad Sci 259:7–16, 1975.
6. Smith CJ, Kelleher RC: αfetoprotein: separation of two molecular variants by affinity chromatography with concanavalin-A agarose. Biochim Biophys Acta 317:231–235, 1973.
7. Abelev GI, Perova S, Khramkova NI, Postnikova ZA, Irlin I: Production of embryonal alphaglobulin by the transplantable mouse hepatomas. Transplant Bull 1:174–180, 1963.
8. Tatarinov YS: Detection of embryospecific alphaglobulin in the blood serum of patients with primary liver tumour. Vopr Med Khim 10:90–91, 1964.
9. Nørgaard-Pederson B, Albrechtsen R, Teilum G: Serum alphafetoprotein as a marker for endodermal sinus tumour (yolk sac tumour) or a vitelline component of teratocarcinoma. Acta Pathol Microbiol Scand 83:573–589, 1975.
10. Talerman A, Haije WG: Alphafetoprotein and germ cell tumours: a possible role of yolk sac tumour in production of alphaprotein. Cancer 34:1722–1726, 1974.
11. Teilum G: Endodermal sinus tumours of the ovary and testis. Comparitive morphogenesis of the so-called mesonephroma ovarii (Schiller) and extra embryonic (yolk sac allantoic) structures of the rat placenta. Cancer 12:1092–1105, 1959.
12. Rosen SW: Placental proteins and their subunits as tumour markers. Ann Intern Med 82:71–83, 1975.
13. Catalona WJ, Vaitukaitis JL, Fair WR: Falsely positive specific human chorionic gonadotrophin assays in patients with testicular tumours: conversion to negative with testosterone administration. J Urol 122:126–128, 1979.
14. Burtin B, Gold P: Carcinoembryonic antigen. Scand J Immunol 8 (Suppl. 8):27–38, 1978.
15. Goldenberg DM: Introduction to the International Conference on the Clinical applications of CEA, Lexington Kentucky 1977. Cancer 42:1397–1398, 1977.
16. Banwo O, Versey J, Hobbs JR: New oncofetal antigen for human pancreas. Lancet i:643–645, 1974.
17. Knapp ML, Hobbs JR: Oncofetal pancreatic antigen. Protides of the Biologic Fluids 27:63–66, 1980.

18. Searle F: New marker possibilities, pp 233-249. In: Germ cell tumours, Anderson, Jones, Milford Ward (eds). London: Taylor & Francis, 1981.
19. Medical Research Council: Myelomatosis: comparison of melphalan and cyclophosphamide therapy. Br Med J 1:640-641, 1971.
20. Axellson U, Hallan JA: A population study on monoclonal gammopathy. Acta Med Scand, 191:111-113, 1972.
21. Kohn J, Shrivastava PC: Paraproteinaemia in blood donors and the aged: benign and malignant. Protides of the Biologic Fluids 20:257-261, 1972.
22. Gutman AB, Gutman EB: Acid phosphatase occurring in serum of patients with metastasising carcinoma of the prostate gland. J Clin Invest 17:473-478, 1938.
23. Foti AG, Herschman H, Cooper JT: A solid phase RIA for human prostatic acid phosphatase. Cancer Res 35:2446-2452, 1975.
24. Huggins C, Hodges CT: Studies on prostatic acid phosphatase I. The effect of castration, of oestrogen, and of androgen injection on serum acid phosphatase in metastatic carcinoma of prostate. Cancer Res 1:293-297, 1941.
25. Cooper EH, Milford Ward A: Acute phase reactant proteins as aids to monitoring disease. Invest Cell Pathol 2:293-301, 1979.
26. Milford Ward A, Cooper EH, Turner R, Anderson JA, Neville AM: Acute phase reactant protein profiles: an aid to the monitoring of large bowel cancer by carcinoembryonic antigen and serum enzymes. Br J Cancer 35:170-178, 1977.
27. Milford Ward A, Cooper EH, Houghton AL: Acute phase reactant proteins in prostatic cancer. Br J Urol 49:411-418, 1977.
28. Te Velde ER, Faber JAJ, Roebersen W, Berghuys M, Zegers BJM, Ballieux RE: The predictive value of serial determinations of some acute phase reactants, complement components and immunoglobulins in patients with invasive carcinoma of the cervix. Protides of the Biologic Fluids 27:335-338, 1980.
29. Bradwell AR: Haptoglobin and orosomucoid in lung and breast tumours, pp 197-215. In: Immunochemistry in clinical laboratory medicine, Milford Ward, Whicher (eds). Lancaster: MTP Press, 1979.
30. Bastable JRG, Richards B, Howarth S, Cooper EH: Acute phase reactant proteins in the management of carcinoma of the bladder. Br J Urol 51:283-289, 1979.
31. Latner AL, Turner GA, Lamin MM: Plasma alpha 1 antitrypsin levels in early and late carcinoma of the cervix. Oncology 33:12-14, 1976.
32. Child JA, Cooper EH, Illingworth S, Worthy TS: Biochemical markers in Hodgkin's disease and non-Hodgkin's lymphoma. Recent Results Cancer Res 64:180-189, 1978.
33. Gold P, Freedman SO: Demonstration of tumour specific antigens in human colonic carcinomata by immunological tolerance and absorption techniques. J Exp Med 121:439-462, 1965.
34. Abelev GI: αfetoprotein as a marker of embryo specific differentiations in normal and tumour tissues. Transplant Rev 20:3-37, 1974.
35. McIntire KR, Vogel CR, Princler GL, Patel IR: Serum αfetoprotein as a biochemical marker for hepatocellular carcinoma. Cancer Res 32:1941-1946, 1972.
36. Ruoslahti E, Salaspuro M, Pihko H, Anderson L, Seppala M: Serum αfetoprotein: diagnostic significance in liver disease. Br Med J 2:527-529, 1974.
37. Sizaret P, Tuyns A, Martel N, Jouvencaux A, Levin A, Ong YW, Rive J: αfetoprotein levels in normal males from seven ethnic groups with different hepatocellular carcinoma risks. Ann NY Acad Sci 259:136-155, 1975.
38. Jalanko H, Engvall E, Virtanen I, Ruoslahti E: Early increase of serum αfetoprotein in spontaneous hepatocarcinogenesis in mice. Int J Cancer 21:453-459, 1978.
39. Kroes R, Sontag JM, Sell S, Williams GM, Weisberger JH. Elevated concentrations of serum alphafetoprotein in rats with chemically induced liver tumours. Cancer Res 35:1214-1217, 1975.

40. Murray Lyon IM, Orr AH, Gazzard B, Kohn J, Williams R: Prognostic value of serum alphafetoprotein in fulminant hepatic failure including patients treated by charcoal haemoperfusion. Gut 17:576-580, 1976.
41. Okuda K, Kotoda K, Obata H, Hayashi N, Hisamitsu T, Tamiya M, Kubo Y, Yakushiji F, Nagata E, Jinnouchi S, Shimokawa Y: Clinical observations during a relatively early stage of hepatocellular carcinoma with special reference to αfetoprotein levels. Gastroenterology 69:226-234, 1975.
42. Co-ordinating Group for the Research on Liver Cancer Studies on human αfetoprotein I. αfetoprotein assay in primary hepatocellular carcinoma. Mass survey and followup studies, The Peoples Republic of China, 1974.
43. McIntire KR, Waldmann TA, Moertel CG, Go VLW: Serum αfetoprotein as a biochemical marker for the gastrointestinal tract. Cancer Res 35:991-996, 1975.
44. Kohn J: The dynamics of serum alphafetoprotein in the course of testicular teratoma. Scand J Immunology 8 (Suppl. 8):103-107, 1978.
45. Lange PH, Fraley EE: Serum alphafetoprotein and testicular tumours. N Engl J Med 296:694, 1977.
46. Bagshawe KD: Choriocarcinoma. London: Arnold, 1969.
47. Bagshawe KD: Recent observations related to the chemotherapy and immunology of gestational choriocarcinoma. Adv Cancer Res 18:231-263, 1973.
48. Bagshawe KD, Harland S: Immunodiagnosis and monitoring of gonadotrophin producing metastases in the central nervous system. Cancer 38:112-118, 1976.
49. Newlands ES, Dent J, Kardona A, Searle F, Bagshawe KD: Serum αfetorprotein and hCG in patients with testicular tumours. Lancet ii:744-745, 1976.
50. Milford Ward A: Markers in germ cell tumours: the current state of the art, AFP, βHCG and AHL kinetics, pp 207-215. In: Germ cell tumours, Anderson, Jones, Milford Ward (eds). London: Taylor and Francis, 1981.
51. Javadpour N: Management of seminoma based as tumour markers. Urol Clin North Am 7:773-780, 1980.
52. Jones WG: Germ cell tumours - the current state of the art and problems in clinical management, pp 3-14. In: Germ cell tumours, Anderson, Jones, Milford Ward (eds). London: Taylor and Francis, 1981.
53. Wiltshaw E: Germ cell tumours in females, pp 179-188. In: Germ cell tumours, Anderson, Jones, Milford Ward (eds). London: Taylor and Francis, 1981.
54. Corbett PJ: Extragonadal germ cell tumours: biological and clinical relevance, pp 165-168. In: Germ cell tumours, Anderson, Jones Milford Ward (eds). London: Taylor and Francis, 1981.
55. Milford Ward A, Bates GE: Serum AFP and apparent half life estimates in the management of endodermal sinus tumours. Protides of the Biologic Fluids 27:356-368, 1980.
56. Javadpour N: Improved staging for testicular cancer using biologic tumour markers: a prospective study. J Urol 124:58-59, 1980.
57. Scott IV, Milford Ward A, Bradwell AR, Wilson A: αfetoprotein, HCG apparent half life in the clinical management of malignant ovarian teratoma, pp 189-191. In Germ cell tumours, Anderson, Jones, Milford Ward (eds). London: Taylor and Francis, 1981.
58. Germa-Lluch JR, Begent RHJ, Bagshawe KD: Tumour marker levels and prognosis in malignant teratoma of the testis. Br J Cancer 42:850-855, 1980.
59. Newlands ES, Begent RHJ, Kaye SB, Rustin GJS, Bagshawe KD: Chemotherapy of advanced malignant teratoma. Br J Cancer 42:378-384, 1980.
60. Begent RHJ, Newlands ES, Germa-Lluch JK, Bagshawe KD: Tumour marker levels and prognosis in malignant teratoma of the testis, pp 227-229. In: Germ cell tumours, Anderson, Jones, Milford Ward (eds). London: Taylor & Francis, 1981.
61. Einhorn LH, Donohue JP: Cisdiammine-dichloroplatinum, vinblastine, and bleomycin

combination chemotherapy in disseminated testicular cancer. Ann Intern Med 87:293–298, 1977.

62. Newlands ES, Begent RHJ, Rustin GJS, Bagshawe KD: The development of modern chemotherapy for malignant teratomas and results of sequential chemotherapy at Charing Cross Hospital, pp 359–367. In: Germ cell tumours, Anderson, Jones, Milford Ward (eds). London: Taylor & Francis, 1981.
63. Hancock BW, Grail A, Bates GE, Jones WG, Milford Ward A: Serum ferritin as a third marker in malignant germ cell tumours, pp 253–255. In: Germ cell tumours, Anderson, Jones, Milford Ward (eds). London: Taylor & Francis, 1981.
64. National Institutes of Health, Concensus Development Conference Statement: CEA: its role as a marker in the management of cancer. Tumour Diagnostik 2:59–61, 1981.
65. Livingstone AS, Hampson LG, Shuster J, Gold P, Hinchley EJ: Carcinoembryonic antigen in the diagnosis and management of colorectal carcinoma. Arch Surg 109:259–264, 1974.
66. Neville AM, Patel S, Lawrence DJR, Cooper EH, Tuberville C, Coombes RC: The monitoring role of plasma CEA alone and in association with other tumour markers in colorectal and mammary carcinoma. Cancer 42:1448–1451, 1978.
67. Sugarbaker PH, Zamcheck N, Moore FD: Assessment of serial carcinoembryonic assays in postoperative detection of recurrent colorectal carcinoma. Cancer 38:2310–2315, 1976.
68. MRC Working Party: Report on the second myelomatosis trial after five years follow-up. Br J Cancer 42:813–822, 1980.
69. MRC Working Party: Prognostic features in the third MRC myelomatosis trial. Br J Cancer 42:831–840, 1980.

4. Biochemical Changes

M. A. PRENTON

1. Biochemical markers of tumour response

Subsequent chapters will concentrate specifically on hormonal markers and endocrine-metabolic measurements and on protein-polypeptide tumour markers; in this chapter a variety of other biochemical markers will be discussed, those whose measurement generally falls within the province of the clinical chemist.

One of the difficulties of reviewing published work on the use of biochemical markers in monitoring effectiveness of treatment is that the majority of studies have concentrated on the value of these markers in diagnosis of tumours. In this context the test must be highly sensitive and specific to the tumour concerned. In monitoring progress of disease and the effect of treatment, however, what matters in the individual patient is that the marker is present and that its level reflects some aspect of tumour activity. Markers only moderately frequently present and thus not suitable for diagnostic purposes may nevertheless be most useful indices of activity in patients in whom they are present. The biochemical measurements discussed may accordingly not have been examined directly in the context of monitoring therapy, but in each case there is evidence that their levels reflect tumour mass or activity. Their potential value in assessment of response may require appropriately designed further study.

Having chosen a suitable marker, the investigator must collect the necessary information to decide the quantity of change in the level of the marker which can be reliably ascribed to a change in the mass or activity of tumour. This requires knowledge of the expected variation between two samples taken at an interval sufficiently short to exclude tumour change; this variation contains both patient and laboratory factors. Ideally, some independent assessment of tumour size, of well documented accuracy, should be simultaneously made.

The tests discussed below have been grouped into those which appear directly to reflect tumour mass, and those which reflect the presence and extent of metastasis in specific sites. It may be worth reminding the reader unfamiliar with laboratory work that care is necessary when comparing published results of enzyme assays with those from one's own laboratory. Variation in normal values for these assays can be extremely wide; many

Hancock, B. W. (ed.), Assessment of Tumour Response.
 ISBN 90-247-2712-X.
Printed in The Netherlands.

publications quote neither the measurement temperature nor the normal limits. When the latter are given it is safest to compare values in terms of multiples of the upper limits.

2. Indices related directly to change in tumour burden

Several aspects of the difference in behaviour of tumour cells may be exploited in applying assays of biochemical markers to assess the total mass of neoplastic cells. Enzymes and metabolites normally mainly located intracellularly are released on cell death: many tumours have a greater cell-loss factor than normal tissues [1] and release rates are correspondingly high. Metabolic pathways related to rapid growth are accentuated in neoplasia, magnifying the changes in the components released: increased catabolism of carbohydrates and anabolism of proteins are examples. These changes lead to a general similarity in tissue enzyme patterns in tumours despite various origins [2].

Tumours arising in some specialised tissues generate metabolites of high specificity which may be measured. Similarly, a few tissues exhibit an enzyme or isoenzyme composition sufficiently specific to allow monitoring of neoplastic growth.

2.1. Tumour mass-related indices of low specificity

Measurements in this category which have been advocated for tumour activity monitoring include several enzymes widely distributed in tissues, certain isoenzymes found in a variety of neoplasms, and more recently, the polyamine group of metabolites. Though their low specificity severely limits use of these markers in *diagnosis* of neoplasms, an elevated level which can be reliably ascribed to the presence of a known tumour can closely reflect the activity of growth and accordingly the response to therapy.

Elevated serum levels of several enzymes of carbohydrate metabolism can be demonstrated in patients with a variety of tumours. The two most often applied to monitoring of neoplastic activity are glucosephosphate isomerase (GPI), also known as phosphohexose isomerase, and lactate dehydrogenase (LDH).

The methodology for GPI was defined [3] and the enzyme used as an index of metastatic breast carcinoma growth [4] over twenty-five years ago. The serum activity has been shown to be more often elevated than other carbohydrate metabolizing enzymes in patients with carcinomas of breast [5], gastrointestinal tract [6], head, neck and oesophagus [7], and lung [8]. Similar results were found in a study [9] of 284 patients with liver metastases from a variety of primary carcinomas. Griffith and Beck assessed the value of GPI in monitoring metastatic breast cancer activity [10]: changes in activity always corresponded with other measures of disease progress, and seemed more reliable than changes in serum and urine calcium. Levels were normal in carcinomas without detectable spread beyond the breast; similar results were found for other localised cancers. Schwarz *et al.* [11] in studies of four cases of advanced prostatic cancer, found GPI correlated better with exacerbations of the disease than did levels of acid phosphatase. The enzyme has been found to be of comparable value to carcinoembryonic antigen, gamma-glutamyl transferase and LDH in monitoring cancer activity [12].

GPI may be elevated in several clinical situations other than disseminated malignancy. These are mainly hepatic disorders, particularly hepatitis, but to a lesser extent biliary obstruction; major surgery may cause elevations persisting up to ten days, possibly accentuated by blood transfusion.

Elevated LDH activity in serum in association with neoplasia was first demonstrated by Hill and Levi [13] in 1954, who found abnormal levels in 48 of 51 patients. In studies where GPI has also been measured [5–9] LDH is usually elevated somewhat less frequently than the isomerase. However, it is an enzyme commonly measured on a routine basis, often as part of a 'biochemical profile', and its greater availability may be an advantage. In one of the small number of recent reports of the application of LDH assay, Bosl *et al.* [14] compared the enzyme with human chorionic gonadotrophin (HCG), alphafetoprotein (AFP) and carcinoembryonic antigen (CEA) in the monitoring of nonseminomatous testicular tumours: LDH performed very comparably with HCG and AFP and other measures of disease response. CEA did not prove a useful marker in this context.

Awais has suggested that LDH may be a useful marker of ovarian carcinoma activity [15, 16]. Though only small numbers of cases were studied, elevated values were found in virtually 100% and all decreased after tumour resection. In his earlier retrospective study [15] benign ovarian conditions (28 cases) all showed normal levels, as did 16 cases of colon cancer and 22 cases of breast cancer – findings very much at odds with other publications. Burrows [17] studied 61 patients preoperatively: frequency of abnormal results was not cited but mean values for both localised and metastatic ovarian cancers were within the normal range, suggesting a much lower level of sensitivity than found by Awais. Though neither author's findings lend much support to the diagnostic application of the assay, its use in monitoring disease progress and response perhaps merits further examination in this group of tumours. Several conditions other than changing tumour burdens lead to raised LDH levels. Those most likely to lead to problems of interpretation in this context are acute or chronic liver disease, folate deficiency and perhaps cancer-associated myopathy.

Isoenzymes of LDH have been studied in neoplastic tissue by several groups of workers [18, 19]; though most cancers contain mainly LDH-3,4 and 5, this has not been reflected in serum levels, probably because of the different disappearance rates of the isoenzymes. This, together with the increased technical effort of isoenzyme measurements, seriously limits their use in tumour activity monitoring.

A number of other enzymes and isoenzymes which may prove to be of value in monitoring tumour activity have been identified in serum in association with neoplasms. The first of the placental-like isoenzymes of alkaline phosphatase was named by Fishman [20], the Regan isoenzyme after the patient in whose bronchial carcinoma it was found. Two other named variants, the Nagas [21] and Regan Variant [22] have been described, but it is clear that many different isoenzymes with the characteristics of placental alkaline phosphatase may occur [23]. There is some evidence that serum measurement may be a useful index of tumour burden [24, 25]. Although the proportion of patients with measurable levels ranges from five to twenty per cent only, the placental isoenzyme is easily measured by standard laboratory methods with minor chemical modifications, and could well be of practical value in these selected patients.

More recently, another isoenzyme of alkaline phosphatase, named the fast homoarginine-sensitive alkaline phosphatase because of its electrophoretic mobility and inhibition characteristics, has been shown to be present in the sera of a large proportion of patients with carcinomas of lung and pancreas [26]. If a correlation between serum activity and tumour burden is confirmed, this assay may be a further addition to the range of useful enzyme markers of disease response.

The value of assay of arylsulphatase, a lysosomal enzyme, in the urine of patients with colorectal cancer has been assessed by Morgan and co-workers [27]. Elevated urine outputs were found in over 80% of patients with Dukes' grade C or D lesions, with progressively lower values in grades B and A. Ten of 13 patients who responded to 5-fluorouracil therapy had initially elevated values, and of these eight had distinct falls in urinary output of the enzyme.

There are preliminary reports of the association with breast carcinoma patients of elevated serum levels of an isoenzyme of creatine kinase, distinct from the isoenzymes normally occurring in plasma, which disappears after mastectomy [28, 29]. What appears to be the same isoenzyme was also reported in the serum of a patient with extensive liver metastases from an uncertain primary site. It is believed that the isoenzyme is of mitochondrial origin, so that death or extensive injury to cells ought to be required for its release.

A novel class of non-specific markers of rapid tissue growth, the polyamines, has aroused considerable interest not only as a potential tool for assessing therapeutic response but because the importance of these simple molecules in the physiology of tissue growth is only currently being realised.

The relevance of polyamine measurements in cancer patients has been reviewed by Russell [30], who first reported increased urinary excretion of putrescine, spermidine and spermine (Fig. 1) in these patients [31]. These compounds are produced in proportion to the rate of growth in both normal and neoplastic cells. The concentrations seen in plasma and urine of cancer subjects are related to both high intracellular levels and death of cells, whether due to the intrinsically higher fractional loss mentioned earlier or to successful tumour therapy [30, 32].

$NH_2CH_2CH_2CH_2CH_2NH_2$

Putrescine

$NH_2CH_2CH_2CH_2NHCH_2CH_2CH_2CH_2NH_2$

Spermidine

$NH_2CH_2CH_2CH_2NHCH_2CH_2CH_2CH_2NHCH_2CH_2CH_2NH_2$

Spermine

Figure 1. Structure of polyamines of importance in mammalian cells.

Until recently polyamines were regarded as excretory products or the end result of tissue putrefaction. This view now holds only for cadaverine, which is formed from lysine by bacterial activity. The role of these compounds remains incompletely understood, but they undoubtedly participate in cellular proliferation and appear to be essential factors in DNA replication and RNA and protein synthesis [33].

Perhaps the major potential importance of polyamine measurements is their ability to give a rapid indication of response to a particular chemotherapeutic regime [34, 35]. Successful therapy is marked by an early rise in urine spermidine excretion. A somewhat later rise in putrescine may predict patients who will fail to respond. Pretreatment levels which become normal after a course of chemotherapy may be an indication of remission. Information of this kind is available much earlier than bone marrow or radiological examination, and promises to be invaluable in tumours difficult to assess by more conventional means.

Measurements of polyamines have been studied in a wide variety of tumours: their application in haematological malignancies has been recently reviewed in detail [36]. Most studies have used urine or plasma measurements, but a recent publication [37] has underlined the value of cerebrospinal fluid polyamine assays in predicting recurrence of medulloblastoma.

Desser [36] has also examined the available data on effects of physiological variables on these estimations, and their derangements in non-malignant diseases. Some of these variations, such as the male: female differences, would not affect the application under consideration, since differences between pre- and post-treatment levels only are relevant. However, fluctuations in spermidine and spermine during the menstrual cycle and the elevated levels of spermidine and putrescine during pregnancy could influence interpretation in female patients. Non-neoplastic disorders producing raised amounts of polyamines include viral and bacterial infections, various autoimmune disorders such as rheumatoid arthritis, psoriasis, ulcerative colitis, systemic lupus, various anaemias, cystic fibrosis and acromegaly. In many of these conditions short-term variations may well be relatively small and therefore interfere little with interpretation of changes induced by chemotherapy or other treatment.

The main current limitations to wider clinical use of polyamine assays are the relatively lengthy analytical procedure, and equipment required for numerous and precise estimations. In urine the great majority of excreted polyamine is conjugated and requires several hours' hydrolysis before analysis; concentrations of free polyamines in plasma, cerebrospinal fluid and urine are around one-fiftieth of those of the conjugates. Amino-acid analysers or high performance liquid chromatographs, essential for these assays, are now available in the great majority of major clinical centres, however. The development of more sensitive methods, probably immunological, for the lower levels of unconjugated polyamines may be expected to lead to increasing applications of these measurements [38].

2.2. High-specificity indices of tumour burden

The tumours of highly specialised tissues in which measurements or detection of relatively specific enzymes or metabolites have been successfully applied include prostatic carcinoma, the sympathoblastoma group, and melanoma.

In the diagnosis of metastasizing prostatic cancer, serum acid phosphatase assay has been used for forty years or more, since the early work of Gutman and co-workers [39]. Acid phosphatase enzyme activity in serum may have several sources including red cells, white cells and platelets: methods of measurement based on enzyme activity usually employ some means of increasing prostate-specificity, by incorporating inhibitors such as tartrate or using particular substrates such as thymolphthalein phosphate [40]. More recently, highly sensitive immunoassay using antibodies specific to prostatic acid phosphatase have been applied to the early diagnosis of prostatic carcinoma. These developments have been the subject of several appraisals [41-43]. However, although the frequency of abnormalities and the amount of immunoassayable enzyme in the circulation increase parallel with tumour extent, publication of assessment of the value of these newer techniques in monitoring tumour response to treatment is awaited. On present evidence it seems likely that the simpler enzyme-activity techniques, which yield fewer false positive results [42] and have adequate sensitivity in stages of the disease where chemotherapy is applied, may be more practical.

A few recent reports have suggested that the isoenzyme of creatine kinase normally associated with brain tissue (CK-BB) might be useful as a marker of prostatic carcinoma. The low incidence in patients with the disease, and difficulties of interpretation caused by release of the enzyme from other sites in the urinary tract as a result of infection or obstruction, make this assay unlikely to be helpful in assessing therapeutic response [44].

The group of tumours collectively referred to as sympathoblastomas includes phaeochromocytomas, neuroblastomas, ganglioneuromas and retinoblastomas. They arise from tissues with embryonic origins in the neural crest. Melanomas share this common origin and both groups of tissues rely on metabolism of the phenolic amino acids phenylalanine and tyrosine for the generation of their major functional molecules, the catecholamines noradrenaline and adrenaline, and melanin. The shared biosynthetic pathways are briefly summarised in Fig. 2. The enzymic conversion of dopamine to noradrenaline is relevant to the choice of metabolite for monitoring of tumour activity, since in relatively poorly differentiated neuroblastomas and malignant phaeochromocytomas, dopamine β-hydroxylase is deficient, leading to excretion of dopa (dihydroxyphenylalanine) and its metabolite vanillactic acid (VLA) rather than homovanillic (HVA) and vanilmandelic (VMA) acids [45, 46].

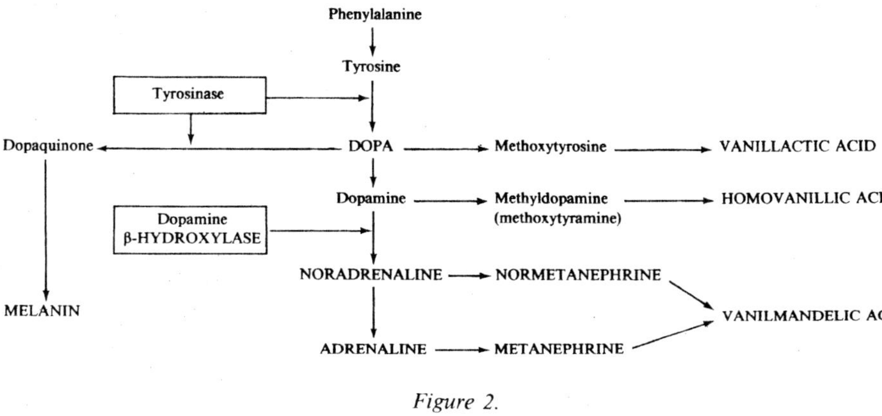

Figure 2.

The great majority of patients with neuroblastoma, ganglioneuroblastoma and ganglioneuroma excrete increased amounts of HVA and VMA. LaBrosse *et al.* [47] found elevated values of HVA in 75% and of VMA in 71% of cases examined in a study of 288 patients. Laug *et al.* [46] found elevations of one or both metabolites in 51 of 54 cases examined before treatment. Other metabolites studied by the latter authors in the same group of patients showed increased VLA in 22% and 3-methoxytyrosine in 22%. In a limited study of dopa excretion, Türler and Käser [45] found elevated values in all 12 cases of neuroblastoma studied. Measurements of HVA and VMA are, however, more widely available and therefore of more practical value.

Another metabolite, cystathionine, has been suggested as a marker of activity of these tumours. This intermediate of methionine metabolism is a normal constituent of neural tissue and not otherwise found in urine except in the rare inherited disease of cystathioninuria, and has been reported in a few cases of hepatoblastoma. Geiser and Efron [48] found elevations in 50 per cent of 28 patients with active neuroblastoma or ganglioneuroblastoma, with no false positive findings. Normal values were found in successfully treated cases. Laug *et al.* [46] found cystathioninuria in 57 per cent of their cases, mainly in those with disseminated disease.

Using measurements of HVA and VMA, Liebner and Rosenthal [49] were able to show in a study of 16 children with neuroblastoma, good correlation with effective treatment, and results of initiating further treatment on the basis of biochemical evidence alone were encouraging. Guitterez Moyano *et al.* [50] were able to follow 31 children after treatment using VMA and noradrenaline excretion: all but one of fourteen patients whose results became normal after treatment were apparently cured (after 1–4 years), while all other seventeen cases were either dead or had advanced disease.

Dopa, the biochemical precursor common to both the catecholamines and melanin, was found by Voorhess [51] to be the metabolite most often excreted in excess by patients with advanced melanoma. Of the 16 cases studied, 14 had melanotic tumours: of these, seven had elevated dopa in urine. Several other markers were studied, including dopamine, HVA, noradrenaline, adrenaline and VMA, each being elevated in three or four cases. Five individuals and one of the amelanotic cases had no demonstrable abnormality; the remaining amelanotic patient showed a slight excess of dopamine only. In a larger study, Hinterberger *et al.* [52] measured urinary dopa, dopamine and dihydroxyphenyl-acetic acid. Only one of 22 cases with stages II–IV disease had normal dopa excretion: the other metabolites were less frequently abnormal. Higher levels of metabolites were found in urine of patients with more widespread disease. No information was given in this report about presence or absence of pigment in the tumours.

Other groups have confirmed the usual absence of these metabolites in patients with amelanotic tumours, which is related to the near-zero activity of the tyrosinase-dopa oxidase enzyme complex (Fig. 2) in the tissue. The low activity found in some melanotic tumours may explain the absence of increased metabolite excretion in some (but not all) of those patients. Morgan and co-workers [53] found that HVA was increased above control values in 13 of 19 melanotic but also in 7 of 19 amelanotic cases, even though dopa oxidase activity in tumour tissue in the latter group was uniformly low.

In contrast with the above measurements of specific metabolites, Pavel and others [54] have recently described the application of a simple colorimetric test, originally described in 1937 [55] for the determination of dopa, to the urine of a patient with melanoma. The reaction is positive for several o-dihydroxy compounds including dopa and 5-hydroxyindoles, and in view of its simplicity deserves further assessment of its clinical value in disseminated melanoma and its therapy.

The tumours of prostate and tissues of neural crest origin which have been discussed appear to be exceptional in their production of relatively easily measured biochemical markers of relatively high specificity (if one excludes hormonal markers, discussed in another chapter). The claim that high gamma glutamyl transferase activity in ascitic fluid in hepatocellular carcinoma is specific [56] is not substantiated, being equally raised in subjects with alcoholic cirrhosis [57, 58]. Hada *et al.* have characterised a novel isoenzyme of gamma glutamyl transferase in tumour tissue in 5 of 10 patients with renal carcinoma [59], but the presence of usefully measurable levels of the isoenzyme in plasma have yet to be assessed.

3. Indices of metastases

The potential importance of markers of the presence of metastases in assessing therapeutic effect is twofold: appearance of metastases implies escape from or failure of the treatment regime, and secondly, rising or falling levels of indicator molecules may be expected to relate to the effects on specific organs of growth or quantity of tumour tissue with them. Because of its fundamental influence on choice of initial treatment of the cancer patient, methods for detection of the presence of metastases have been extensively studied. The liver and the skeleton are of course the organs whose involvement by tumour results in the appearance of circulating markers of adequate specificity and sensitivity.

3.1. Indices of hepatic metastases

The efficacy of any pre-mortem method for detecting metastatic disease in the liver is substantially less than perfect. Even palpation of the liver at laparotomy has been shown to miss around 5 per cent [60] to 8 per cent [61] of deposits detected by careful postmortem examination. Evaluation of the diagnostic efficiency of biochemical markers of liver metastases must accordingly take into account the diagnostic reference method used.

The study of Kim *et al.* [62] of consecutive untreated patients used mainly isotope scanning, in combination with echograms and liver biopsy in some patients. The serum activities of alkaline phosphatase (ALP), 5′-nucleotidase (5NT), gamma-glutamyl transferase (GGT) and glutamate dehydrogenase (GDH) were studied in 95 patients of whom 40 had evidence of metastases, a prevalence of 42 per cent. 5NT was the best predictor of the presence of liver deposits, only 14 per cent of positive results occurring in their absence. The other three enzymes, ALP, GGT and GDH, gave 37 to 42 per cent of abnormal results in the absence of other evidence of deposits in the liver. However, GGT was the best test for excluding metastases, only 3 per cent of tests being normal when deposits were present, compared with 20 to 24 per cent for the other three enzymes.

In the larger series of Beck *et al.* [63] the prevalence of liver metastases by palpation at laparotomy was 17 per cent of 184 cases. Fifty-two per cent had apparently curative resection, the remaining 31 per cent having either extensive local spread, inoperable tumour, or metastases not involving the liver. The enzymes studied in relation to hepatic metastasis were GGT, ALP, 5NT, LDH and glutathione reductase. Though the data are not presented in the same way, the relevant enzyme results can be compared with the study cited above by recalculation. Again, 5NT was better than GGT in predicting the presence of deposits, but both enzymes gave more falsely positive results (57 and 81 per cent) than in the study of Kim *et al.* [62]. Of the other enzymes, ALP was about as good as 5NT. All three enzymes performed similarly in excluding metastases, with 11–12 per cent of normal results in their presence. The apparently inferior overall performance of the tests in this study is partly related to the lower prevalence of metastases in the cases studied. Had the prevalence been 42 per cent in this study, falsely positive tests for 5NT and GGT would have been 27 and 41 per cent, respectively. This rather confusing effect of variation in prevalence between studies on the apparent performance of tests, has been usefully discussed by Vecchio [64]. Awareness of the phenomenon is essential to reliable comparison between published work and one's own practice. The other important difference between the two studies is the method of detection of metastases; a better correlation of enzyme tests with positive liver scanning than with laparotomy diagnosis might be due to easier detection of smaller or fewer deposits by the latter technique.

In a recently published study of patients with lymphoma [65], 9 of 72 patients (13 per cent) were judged to have hepatic involvement by isotope scan and biopsy 'where appropriate'. At initial examination all nine patients had abnormal 5NT and eight abnormal ALP values, compared with respectively 9 and 15 of the 63 patients apparently free of liver deposits. These results translate into false positive rates of 50 per cent for 5NT and 65 per cent for ALP, and corresponding false negative frequencies of 0 and 2 per cent. Extrapolation of the data to a prevalence similar to that found by Kim *et al.* would reduce the false negative rates for 5NT to 16 per cent and for ALP to 27 per cent, results little different from that study.

In each of these investigations, measurements of the enzymes currently believed to be the most sensitive and specific for the purpose do not have the predictive power most clinicians would require for decisions affecting therapy. Improved performance may result if combinations of tests are used, provided they are selected so that their sequential application screens out the cases without metastasis, so as to increase progressively the prevalence of secondary tumour cases to which the more specific tests are applied. Further appropriately designed studies are required before these measurements can be of real practical value in guiding treatment.

3.2. *Indices of bone metastases*

Of the biochemical markers easily measured for the assessment of bone metastatic disease, serum alkaline phosphatase activity and urine hydroxyproline are the most frequently used.

Though alkaline phosphatase is widely measured as an index of metastasis to both bone and liver, there have been few published studies of its application in monitoring response to treatment. Part of the reason may be the technical difficulty of separate assessment of the activities of the bone and liver isoenzymes. Total enzyme activity may also be rather insensitive to the presence of bone deposits; in studies of breast [66] and lymphoid [65] malignancy, only half of those patients with radiological evidence of osseous disease had elevated levels. In a large series of patients with proven bone metastasis from prostatic cancer [67], however, 85 per cent showed elevated total activity; a further 7 per cent (with normal total activity) could be shown to have increases of the bone isoenzyme. In the latter study, results from a subgroup of 105 patients were examined for correlation with clinical response to treatment: 68 failed to respond, 31 became stable and 6 showed a partial response. These groups had significantly different mean initial levels of total and bone alkaline phosphatase, high levels predicting failure of response. Of 46 patients whose enzyme levels were measured at the time of assessing response, 22 failed to respond, 19 were 'stable' and 5 showed a partial response. Applying the criterion of a less than 25 per cent fall in enzyme activity from the initial level as a test to predict progression, this was correct on 63 per cent of occasions for total enzyme and 70 per cent for bone isoenzyme, a false-positive rate of about one-third.

The hydroxyproline of urine is mainly derived from the breakdown of recently formed collagen and is consequently a useful index of the rate of bone turnover. Increases above normal adult levels are found in association with the rapid bone growth of childhood and adolescence, and in conditions such as hyperparathyroidism, hyperthyroidism and Paget's disease, as well as with the presence of certain metastatic tumours in bone [68, 69]. Male subjects have greater daily excretion values than females. The contribution from the diet to the urine output can be virtually eliminated by a short period of restriction.

Cuschieri [66] studied 47 cases of breast cancer including 12 with radiologically demonstrable skeletal deposits, 9 who developed them during the study, 10 with soft-tissue deposits only and 18 with localised disease. Only the first two groups had elevations of urine hydroxyproline at the start, and sequential examinations showed that increases in output predated X-ray appearance of metastases by several months. This study unfortunately gives no information on the sensitivity or specificity of hydroxyproline measurements in this context.

Pandya and others [70] compared the relative values of hydroxyproline and CEA, and reported a sensitivity of 58 per cent in breast cancer with osseous metastases. The criterion for diagnosis of the deposits was not stated. The presentation of the data does not allow proper assessment of specificity, though no elevated values were found amongst 62 tests on an unstated number of 'post-mastectomy disease-free patients'. The authors concluded that the test was insensitive but specific in comparison to CEA measurement. Deeble and Goldberg [65], in their two-year follow-up study of 72 lymphoma patients, also demonstrated the greater sensitivity of hydroxyproline than X-rays in detection of skeletal involvement. These authors found 24 patients with raised hydroxyproline excretion, 20 of which had or later developed evidence of bone disease (radiology, marrow biopsy and bone scintiscanning). When the hydroxyproline excretion was 'corrected' for urine creatinine (a procedure recommended by most earlier authors) four additional patients had elevated levels, increasing the 'false-positive' rate from 17 to 29 per cent. In contrast to the study mentioned earlier on breast cancer patients, all patients with demonstrable bone deposits of lymphoma gave raised hydroxyproline values.

4. Conclusions

From the observations made at the beginning of this chapter it will be clear that practical application of the majority of the biochemical markers discussed is hampered by lack of precise information upon the relation between changes in marker level and tumour activity, or well-defined estimates of the predictive value of a positive test for presence of metastasis. Reliable evaluation of new forms of therapy, or proper support for clinical decisions to modify treatment of the individual patient, will require considerable further study.

References

1. Steel GG: Cell loss as a factor in the growth rate of human tumours. Eur J Cancer 3:381–387, 1967.
2. Greenstein JP: Biochemistry of cancer, 2nd ed. New York: Academic Press, 1954.
3. Bodansky O: Serum phosphohexose isomerase in cancer: I, method of determination and establishment of range of normal values. Cancer 7:1191–1199, 1954.
4. Bodansky O: Serum phosphohexose isomerase in cancer: II, as index of tumour growth in metastatic carcinoma of breast. Cancer 7:1200–1226, 1954.
5. Rose A, West M, Zimmerman HJ: Serum enzymes in disease. V. Isocitric dehydrogenase, malic dehydrogenase and glycolytic enzymes in patients with carcinoma of the breast. Cancer 14:726–733, 1961.
6. Schwartz MA, West M, Walsh WS, Zimmerman HJ: Serum enzymes in disease. VIII. Glycolytic and oxidative enzymes and transaminases in patients with gastrointestinal carcinoma. Cancer 15:346–353, 1962.
7. Schwartz MA, Walsh WS, West M, Zimmerman HJ: Serum enzymes in disease. X. Glycolytic and oxidative enzymes and transaminases in patients with carcinomas of the head, neck and oesophagus. Cancer 15:927–930, 1962.
8. West M, Schwartz MA, Walsh WS, Zimmerman HJ: Serum enzymes in disease. XI. Glycolytic and oxidative enzymes and transaminases in patients with cancer of the lung. Cancer 15:931–935, 1962.
9. Tan CO, Cohen J, West M, Zimmerman HJ: Serum enzymes in disease. XIV. Abnormality of levels of transaminases and glycolytic and oxidative enzymes and of liver functions as related to the extent of metastatic carcinoma of the liver. Cancer 16:1373–1387, 1963.
10. Griffith MM, Beck JC: The value of serum phosphohexose isomerase as an index of metastatic breast carcinoma activity. Cancer 16:1032–1041, 1963.
11. Schwartz MK, Greenberg E, Bodansky O: Comparative values of phosphatases and other serum enzymes in following patients with prostatic carcinoma. Cancer 16:583–594, 1964.
12. Munjal D, Chawla P, Lokich JJ, Zamcheck N: Carcinoembryonic antigen and phosphohexose isomerase, gamma-glutamyl transpeptidase and lactate dehydrogenase levels in patients with and without liver metastases. Cancer 37:1800–1807, 1976.
13. Hill BR, Levi C: Elevation of a serum component in neoplastic disease. Cancer Res 14:513–515, 1954.
14. Bosl GJ, Lange PH, Nochomovitz LE, Goldmann A, Fraley EE, Rosai J, Johnson K, Kennedy BJ: Tumour markers in advanced nonseminomatous testicular cancer. Cancer 47:572–576, 1981.
15. Awais GM: Serum lactic dehydrogenase levels in the diagnosis and treatment of carcinoma of the ovary. Am J Obstet Gynecol 116:1053–1057, 1973.
16. Awais GM: Carcinoma of the ovary and serum lactic dehydrogenase levels. Surg Gynecol Obstet 146:893–895, 1978.
17. Burrows S: Serum enzymes in the diagnosis of ovarian malignancy. Am J Obstet Gynecol 137:140–141, 1980.
18. Poznanska-Linde H, Wilkinson JH, Withycombe WA: Lactate dehydrogenase isoenzymes in malignant tissues. Nature (Lond) 209:727–728, 1966.

19. Latner AL, Turner DM, Way SA: Enzyme and isoenzyme studies in preinvasive carcinoma of the cervix. Lancet 2:814–816, 1966.
20. Fishman WH, Inglis NI, Stolbach LL, Krant MJ: A serum alkaline phosphatase isoenzyme of human neoplastic cell origin. Cancer Res 28:150–154, 1968.
21. Nakayama T, Yoshida M, Kitamura M: L-leucine sensitive, heat-stable alkaline phosphatase isoenzyme detected in a patient with pleuritis carcinomatosa. Clin Chim Acta 30:546–548, 1970.
22. Higashino K, Hashinotsume M, Kang K-Y, Takahashi Y, Yamamura Y: Studies on a variant alkaline phosphatase in sera of patients with hepatocellular carcinoma. Clin Chim Acta 40:67–81, 1972.
23. Benham FJ, Povey MS, Harris H: Placental-like alkaline phosphatase in malignant and benign ovarian tumours. Clin Chim Acta 86:201–215, 1978.
24. Stolbach LL, Krant MJ, Fishman WH: Ectopic production of an alkaline phosphatase isoenzyme in patients with cancer. N Engl J Med 281:757–761, 1969.
25. Malkin A, Kellen JA, Lickrish GM, Bush RS: Carcinoembryonic antigen (CEA) and other tumour markers in ovarian and cervical cancer. Cancer 42:1452–1456, 1978.
26. Kahan L, Go VLW, Larson FC: Increased activity in serum of an alkaline phosphatase isoenzyme in cancer: analytical method and preliminary clinical studies. Clin Chem 27:104–107, 1981.
27. Morgan LR, Samuels MS, Thomas W, Krementz ET, Meeker W: Arylsulfatase B in colorectal cancer. Cancer 36:2337–2345, 1975.
28. Yuu H, Takagi Y, Senju O, Hosoya J, Gomi K, Ishii T: Creatine kinase isoenzyme of high relative molecular mass in serum of a cancer patient. Clin Chem 24:2054–2057, 1978.
29. Liu TZ, Shen JT, Shohet SB: Atypical cathode-migrating creatine kinase isoenzyme and human breast carcinoma: a specific marker? Clin Chem 26:1765, 1980.
30. Russell DH: Clinical relevance of polyamines as biochemical markers of tumour kinetics. Clin Chem 23:22–27, 1977.
31. Russell DH: Increased polyamine concentrations in the urine of human cancer patients. Nature New Biol 233:144–145, 1971.
32. Heby O, Andersson G: Tumour cell death: the probable cause of increased polyamine levels in physiological fluids. Acta Path Microbiol Scand A 86:17–20, 1978.
33. Raina A, Eloranta T, Pajula R-L, Mäntyjärv R, Tuomi K: Polyamine in rapidly growing animal tissues, pp 35–49. In: Polyamines in biomedical research, Gaugas JM (ed). Chichester: John Wiley and Sons, 1980.
34. Russell DH, Durie BGM, Salmon SE: Polyamines as markers of success and failure in cancer chemotherapy, Lancet ii:797–799, 1975.
35. Durie BGM, Salmon SE, Russell DH: Polyamines as markers of response and disease activity in cancer chemotherapy. Cancer Res 37:214–221, 1977.
36. Desser H: Polyamines as markers of malignancy in human leukemia and in other heamatological disorders, pp 415–433. In: Polyamines in biomedical research, Gaugas JM (ed). Chichester: John Wiley and Sons, 1980.
37. Marton LF, Edwards MS, Levin VA, Lubich WP, Wilson CB: CSF polyamines: a new and important means of monitoring patients with medulloblastoma. Cancer 47:757–760, 1981.
38. Seiler N: Assay of polyamines in tissues and body fluids, pp 435–461. In: Polyamines in biomedical research, Gaugas JM (ed). Chichester: John Wiley and Sons, 1980.
39. Gutman AB, Gutman EB: An 'acid' phosphatase occurring in the serum of patients with metastasizing carcinoma of the prostate gland. J. Clin Invest 17:473–379, 1938.
40. Roy AV, Brower ME, Hayden JE: Sodium thymolphthalein monophosphate: a new acid phosphatase substrate with greater specificity for the prostate enzyme in serum. Clin Chem 17:1093–1102, 1971.

41. Romas NA, Rose NR Tannenbaum M: Acid phosphatase: new developments. Hum Pathol 10:501–512, 1979.
42. Griffiths JC: Prostate-specific acid phosphatase: re-evaluation of radioimmunoassay in diagnosing prostatic disease. Clin Chem 26:433–436, 1980.
43. Watson RA, Tang DB: The predictive value of prostatic acid phosphatase as a screening test for prostatic cancer. N Engl J Med 303:497–499, 1980.
44. Homburger HA, Miller SA, Jacob GL: Radioimmunoassay of creatine kinase B-isoenzymes in serum of patients with azotemia, obstructive uropathy, or carcinoma of the prostate or bladder. Clin Chem 26:1821–1824, 1980.
45. Türler K, Käser H: Quantitative fluorimetric determination of urinary dopa and its significance for the diagnosis of neural crest tumours. Clin Chim Acta 32:41–51, 1971.
46. Laug WE, Siegel SE, Shaw KNF, Landing B, Baptista J, Gutenstein M: Initial urinary catecholamine metabolite concentrations and prognosis in neuroblastoma. Paediatrics 62:77–83, 1978.
47. LaBrosse EH, Cons-Nougué C, Zucker-J-M, Comoy E, Bohuon C, Lemerle J, Schweisguth O: Urinary excretion of 3-methoxy-4-hydroxymandelic acid and 3-methoxy-4-hydroxyphenylacetic acid by 288 patients with neuroblastoma and related neural crest tumours. Cancer Res 40:1995–2001, 1980.
48. Geiser CF, Efron ML: Cystathioninuria in patients with neuroblastoma or ganglioneuroblastoma. Cancer 22:856–860, 1968.
49. Liebner EJ, Rosenthal IM: Serial catecholamines in the radiation management of children with neuroblastoma. Cancer 32:623–633, 1973.
50. Gutierrez Moyano MB de, Bergadá C, Becú L: Significance of catecholamine excretion in the follow-up of sympathoblastomas. Cancer 27:228–232, 1971.
51. Voorhess ML: Urinary excretion of DOPA and metabolites by patients with melanoma. Cancer 26:146–149, 1970.
52. Hinterberger H, Freedman A, Bartholomew RJ: Precursors of melanin in the blood and urine in malignant melanoma. Clin Chim Acta 39:395–400, 1972.
53. Morgan LR, Lolley D, Maddox B, Samuels MS, Krementz ET: Urine homovanillic acid and tissue dopa oxidase in patients with melanoma. Cancer 33:1601–1606, 1974.
54. Pavel S, Matous B, Donchon J: Simple screening test for estimation of some phenolic and indolic compounds in urine; application to melanoma. J Invest Dermatol 70:197–199, 1978.
55. Arnow LE: Colorimetric determination of the components of 3,4-dihydroxy-phenylalanine-tyrosine mixtures. J Biol Chem 118: 531–537, 1937.
56. Peters TJ, Seymour CA, Wells G, Fakunle F, Neale G: Gamma-glutamyl transferase levels in ascitic fluid and liver tissue from patients with primary hepatoma. Br Med J 1:1576, 1977.
57. Cortés-Rius M, Escoda J, Fusté L, Queraltó JM, Vilardell F: Gamma-glutamyl transferase in ascitic fluid in primary hepatoma. Br Med J 2:1435, 1978.
58. Olsson R, Waldenstrom J: Gamma-glutamyl transferase activity in ascitic fluid in diagnosis of hepatocellular carcinoma. Br Med J 2:830–831, 1979.
59. Hada T, Higashino K, Yamamoto H, Yamamura Y, Matsuda M, Osafune M, Kotake T, Sonoda T: A novel γ-glutamyl transpeptidase in renal carcinoma in comparison with normal kidney enzyme. Clin Chim Acta 85:267–277, 1978.
60. Hogg L, Pack GT: Diagnostic accuracy of hepatic metastases at laparotomy. Arch Surg 72:251–252, 1956.
61. Gray BN: Surgeon accuracy in the diagnosis of liver metastases at laparotomy. Aust NZ J Surg 50:524–526, 1980.
62. Kim NK, Yasmineh WG, Freier EF, Goldman AI, Theologides A: Value of alkaline phosphatase, 5′-nucleotidase, gamma-glutamyltransferase and glutamate dehydrogenase activity

measurements (single and combined) in serum in diagnosis of metastasis to the liver. Clin Chem 23:2034–2038, 1977.
63. Beck PR, Belfield A, Spooner RJ, Blumgart LH, Wood CB: Serum enzymes in colorectal cancer. Cancer 43:1772–1776, 1979.
64. Vecchio TJ: Predictive value of a single diagnostic test in unselected populations. N Engl J Med 274:1171–1173, 1966.
65. Deeble TJ, Goldberg DM: Assessment of biochemical tests for bone and liver involvement in malignant lymphoma patients. Cancer 45:1451–1457, 1980.
66. Cuschieri A: Urinary hydroxyproline excretion in early and advanced breast cancer – a sequential study. Br J Surg 60:800–803, 1973.
67. Wajsman Z, Chu TM, Bross D, Saroff J, Murphy GP, Johnson DE, Scott WW, Gibbons RP, Pront GR, Schmidt JD: Clinical significance of serum alkaline phosphatase isoenzyme levels in advanced prostatic carcinoma. J Urol 119:244–246, 1978.
68. Mosley HF, Taft EG, Oslen DB, Gates S, Beebe R: Hydroxyproline excretion in malignant neoplastic disease. Arch. Intern Med 118:565–571, 1966.
69. Bonadonna G, Merlino HJ, Laird Myers WP, Sonnenberg M: Urinary hydroxyproline and calcium metabolism in patients with cancer. N Engl J Med 275:298–305, 1966.
70. Pandya KJ, Tormey DC, Waalkes TP, Gehrke C, Hansen H, Neifeld J, Harberg J: Hydroxyproline in breast cancer. Proc Am Assoc Cancer Res 20:223, 1979.

5. Hypercalcaemia and Endocrine Syndromes in Cancer

S. TOMLINSON

1. Hypercalcaemia and cancer

1.1. Introduction

Hypercalcaemia in patients with cancer is common. In about 80% of them it is associated with radiologically detectable bony metastases. Bony metastases occur most commonly in patients with cancer of the breast, lung, kidney, thyroid or prostate; cancer of the breast accounts for 70% of patients with malignant hypercalcaemia in this group. The second group of patients with hypercalcaemia consists of those with lymphomas (including leukaemia) and myeloma which account for about 15% of all cases of malignant hypercalcaemia; many of these patients, particularly those with myeloma, will have osteolytic lesions. The smallest group (less than 10%) are those who have solid tumours without radiologically detectable bony metastases.

1.2. Tumours with bone metastases

Breast cancer is the commonest cause of hypercalcaemia in patients with bony metastases and indeed is the most frequent example of a cancer associated with hypercalcaemia. This might, of course, partly reflect familiarity with this complication in breast cancer; moreover, treatment with sex steroids can induce hypercalcaemia in some patients with disseminated mammary neoplasia (see below), so that some of the hypercalcaemia seen in this condition is iatrogenic. Bone metastases are very common in breast cancer; incidences of up to 90% have been reported and hypercalcaemia associated with the metastases occurs in about one-third of these patients [1]. In addition, hypercalcaemia may be precipitated by initiation of hormone therapy and has been reported to occur in up to 50% of patients at varying times after starting treatment in advanced disease [2]. The picture is further complicated by reports of hypercalcaemia associated with the use of Tamoxifen, an antioestrogen, in breast cancer [3]. Nevertheless, it seems reasonable to conclude that bone destruction as a consequence of metastases from the primary tumour is related to the development of hypercalcaemia.

Hancock, B. W. (ed.), Assessment of Tumour Response.
ISBN 90-247-2712-X.
Printed in The Netherlands.

Presumably, cells are released from the primary site into the circulation and make their way to bone marrow. They then migrate through sinusoids to endosteal bone surface, possibly under the influence of chemotactic signals. Bone destruction is then caused by direct resorption due to tumour cells and indirect resorption possibly related to interactions between tumour cells and lymphocytes and monocytes that accumulate as part of a cell-mediated immune response [4].

The agent responsible for bone resorption has not been unequivocally identified but some evidence suggests that prostaglandins may be important. For example, in one study, explants of human breast cancer cocultivated with bone caused resorption which in turn was prevented by the prostaglandin synthetase inhibitor, indomethacin [5]. Moreover, patients whose cancers showed no *in vitro* osteolytic activity did not develop bony metastases whereas many of those with osteolytic activity, did [6]. Unfortunately the natural corollary of these studies, that inhibition of prostaglandin synthesis might prove useful in malignant hypercalcaemia, has been disappointing [7].

1.3. Hypercalcaemia in myeloma, lymphoma and leukaemia

Hypercalcaemia may develop in up to 30% of patients with myeloma [4] but it is rare in haematological neoplasms like acute leukaemia, chronic lymphocytic leukaemia and lymphoma in which extensive bone marrow infiltration can occur [8, 9, 10]. It seems likely that the reason for this is that myeloma cells produce a soluble factor which stimulates bone resorption but cells from patients with leukaemia and lymphoma, in general, do not secrete this factor; however, if they do, there may be associated hypercalcaemia [11].

In vitro, the factor produced by myeloma cells stimulates osteoclasts to resorb bone and has been called osteoclast activating factor (OAF). This factor was first described in 1972 [12] as an agent known as a lymphokine produced by lymphocytes when stimulated by phytohaemaglutinin. The studies of Mundy and his colleagues [12] have shown that OAF produced by myeloma cells is similar to the lymphokine produced by normal activated lymphocytes. Interestingly, there appears to be an important relationship between OAF and the other potent resorbers of bone, the prostaglandins. Activated lymphocytes only release OAF in the presence of prostaglandins produced by monocytes; moreover, indomethacin and steroids which inhibit prostaglandin synthesis also inhibit OAF production. Glucocorticosteroids can themselves directly inhibit bone resorption caused by OAF [12].

These findings help to explain the usefulness of drugs like prednisolone in the treatment of hypercalcaemia associated with myeloma.

1.4. *Solid tumours without bony metastases*

Hypercalcaemia can occur in patients without obvious bony metastases, and although this is relatively unusual it is important to remember that such patients may present difficulties in differential diagnosis. In a review of hypercalcaemia in neoplastic disease, 56 of 430 patients had no radiologically detectable metastases [1]. The primary tumours arise most commonly in kidney, lung, ovary and pancreas [13]. There is some evidence that the agent responsible for hypercalcaemia in these cases is a parathyroid hormone-like substance [14, 15, 16]. Clinically and biochemically, however, patients with this so-called pseudo-hyperparathyroidism differ from patients with primary hyperparathyroidism. They have, for example, a tendency to alkalosis rather than acidosis and the hypercalcaemia may be suppressed with corticosteroids. In addition, characteristic bony changes seen in some patients with primary hyperparathyroidism are rarely seen in pseudo-hyperparathyroidism. The evidence that biologically active parathyroid hormone is synthesized and secreted by these tumours is not well documented; much of it is circumstantial or based on conflicting immunoassay data which can be notoriously misleading. That some tumours can produce a humoral agent which causes hypercalcaemia is well established but it seems likely that a parathyroid hormone-like substance is rarely responsible. There is some evidence that one of the bone resorbing agents which can be incriminated in this type of hypercalcaemia is a prostaglandin [17]. The strongest evidence comes from work with animal tumour models in which large amounts of prostaglandin E_1 have been shown to be produced *in vitro* and *in vivo* and further, that hypercalcaemia in tumour-bearing animals can be prevented by treatment with indomethacin [18]. In man, increased plasma concentrations of prostaglandin E_2 have been reported in hypercalcaemic patients with malignant disease [19, 20], and increased concentrations of PGE_M, the major metabolite of the E prostaglandins, have been found in the urine of patients with solid tumours and hypercalcaemia [21.

1.5. *Sex steroids, tamoxifen and hypercalcaemia*

1.5.1. Sex steroids. Hypercalcaemia is common in breast cancer. It may be sufficiently severe to cause symptoms. In a series of 127 patients with breast cancer, 18 developed acute hypercalcaemia associated with increased skeletal pain, anorexia, nausea and vomiting; in 8 of the 18 patients, hypercalcaemia occurred at varying times after starting hormone therapy for advanced disease; six of these patients had received fluoxymesterone and two had received stilbestrol [2]. Hypercalcaemia as a consequence of hormone therapy was first recognised in 1953 when it was found in nine patients in a series of 361 women with advanced breast cancer [22]. Again androgens were responsible in the majority (7 patients) and oestrogens in the minority (2 patients). The complication occurred only in patients with bony metastases. The cause of the hypercalcaemia is not understood but it is possible that oestrogens in some way stimulate tumour cells to produce osteolytic substances.

Unfortunately, hypercalcaemia can be rapidly fatal even when recognised and treated. Moreover, its onset seems to be a sign of a poor prognosis since six of the eight patients treated with hormone therapy who developed this complication survived less than six months; indeed only three of the total of 18 patients in the same series survived more than one year [2].

1.5.2. Tamoxifen. Tamoxifen, an antioestrogen has been used successfully in the treatment of breast cancer for a number of years [23, 24, 25]. In 1977 it was first recognised that hypercalcaemia might be an unwanted side effect of the drug [26]. Further reports indicated that it might occur in a large proportion of patients after initiation of therapy and it was suggested that caution was needed particularly in patients with metatastic osteolytic disease [27]. However, controversy developed on this issue; it now seems that the incidence of tamoxifen-induced hypercalcaemia has been overstated [3]. Nevertheless, the consensus appears to be that tamoxifen can cause hypercalcaemia in patients with widespread skeletal metastases particularly if they have a slightly raised pre-treatment serum calcium [28]. It has even been suggested that such a response may predict long-term tumour regression [29] but as yet there is no firm evidence to support such a conclusion.

1.6. Alteration in serum calcium as an index of response to treatment in cancer

It is not easy to assess whether reduction in serum calcium following treatment for cancer may be a good index of satisfactory tumour response nor is it easy to evaluate recurrence of hypercalcaemia as an index of relapse. This is because, if a patient has symptomatic hypercalcaemia, as well as receiving treatment directed at the neoplasm he may also receive treatment specifically for hypercalcaemia. Myers suggested correction of hypercalcaemia can reflect tumour response to treatment [1]. Although treatment of breast cancer associated with severe hypercalcaemia can be corrected by pituitary ablation, additional therapy is frequently required, such as oral or, rarely, intravenous phosphate. Hypercalcaemia may then be corrected but skeletal metastasis may increase and death subsequently occur without recurrence of hypercalcaemia [2]. The inclusion of mithramycin in combination chemotherapy may be associated not only with correction of hypercalcaemia but also with bone healing in a proportion of patients with disseminated mammary neoplasm [31].

Rapid reductions of serum calcium after radiotherapy, nitrogen mustard, methotrexate or cytosine arabinoside-induced remission have been reported in lymphomas and leukaemias [32]. A patient described by Lokich and Shevitz [33] had a greatly elevated serum calcium associated with a lymphocytic lymphoma and combination chemotherapy with other supportive measures including rehydration rapidly resulted in serum calcium returning to normal. In patients with myeloma, treatment with cytotoxic drugs can result in improvement in hypercalcaemia [34] but clearly, just as in lymphoma and leukaemia there are better assessment indices in myeloma than improvement in or even correction of hypercalcaemia.

In patients who have solid tumours without obvious bony metastases it can be expected that correction of hypercalcaemia will normally be a good index of response to treatment. In a series of cases reported by Powell *et al.* [35], remission of hypercalcaemia occurred in 9/11 patients following tumour resection, irradiation or cytotoxic therapy for pseudo-hyperparathyroidism [35]. Hypercalcaemia recurred in three patients with the appearance of metastases and one patient with recurrence of his reticulum-cell sarcoma. In a larger series of 74 patients analysed by Skrabanek *et al.* [16], treatment of the primary tumour resulted in correction of hypercalcaemia in over 80% of them; curiously, however, even in four cases where metastases were present, hypercalcaemia was corrected by resection of the primary tumour.

Clearly, therefore, the distinction between humoral and metastatic hypercalcaemia may be more apparent than real, particularly when one remembers that the absence of detectable metastases on x-rays does not exclude their presence; in fact bone marrow aspirates are often positive for neoplastic cells in patients with negative x-ray findings.

1.7. Differential diagnosis of hypercalcaemia in malignant disease

Since most patients with cancer who have symptomatic hypercalcaemia will have metastases, the differential diagnosis is not usually difficult [36]. Patients with myelomatosis will have serum and bone marrow abnormalities that usually make the diagnosis relatively easy. Similarly, there are clinical and biochemical features in thyroid disease and in Addison's disease which should prevent confusion with cancer. Paget's disease rarely causes hypercalcaemia except when it is severe and accompanied by immobilisation. The principal diagnostic difficulties arise in distinguishing an occult cancer without evidence of metastases from primary hyperparathyroidism and to a lesser extent, sarcoidosis, vitamin D intoxication and milk alkali syndrome.

Clinically, rapidly progressive, severe hypercalcaemia should alert the physician to the possibility of a malignant tumour. From a biochemical point of view, patients with hypercalcaemia due to cancer often have an alkalosis in contrast to the hyperchloraemic acidosis seen in primary hyperparathyroidism; moreover, malignant hypercalcaemia may be suppressible with steroid treatment whereas hypercalcaemia of hyperparathyroidism without bone disease is usually not suppressible with steroids.

In a situation where the diagnosis remains obscure and delay in treatment may be dangerous it seems reasonable to suggest that a careful exploration of the neck by an experienced surgeon will exclude as far as possible, primary hyperparathyroidism. It should be noted, however, that primary hyperparathyroidism and malignant disease may coexist [37].

2. Hormone syndromes and cancer

2.1. Introduction

Many tumours synthesize and secrete hormones not normally made by the tissue from which the tumour originates. This is called 'ectopic hormone production' and is normally associated with tumours of non endocrine origin. These tumours are of interest not only because they may lead us to a better understanding of embryology, molecular biology and histopathology, but also because the metabolic abnormality associated with a particular tumour may be useful as a diagnostic marker or index of tumour response to treatment. Furthermore, the patient's symptoms may be more a reflection of the metabolic abnormality caused by ectopic hormone secretion than the result of the tumour itself.

It should be borne in mind that the concept of ectopic hormone production can be indistinct since some hormones may be made by a particular tissue even when it is not neoplastic. In some cases it is not absolutely clear whether certain cells synthesize and secrete a particular hormone under normal conditions. Here I shall discuss the most common syndromes generally accepted as a result of ectopic hormone production and in addition describe some conditions in which hormones can be used as tumour markers or in which hormones from tumours cause a definable clinical syndrome.

Why can there be some confusion about endocrine syndromes in cancer and why do a wide variety of apparently unrelated tissues that are not associated normally with secretion of a particular hormone acquire this capacity when they undergo neoplastic transformation? It is helpful to consider the APUD concept which provides some common ground to what at first seems a random process.

2.2. *The APUD concept*

Many of the cells associated with ectopic hormone production share basic ultrastructural and cytochemical features. One of these is the capacity to take up substances like DOPA and 5HT, decarboxylate them and subsequently produce biogenic amines; hence Amine Precursor Uptake and Decarboxylation – with the acronym APUD. These cells are embryogically derived from the neural crest and migrate into many tissues and organs during development. These include the lungs, thyroid, pancreas, gut and adrenal medulla. Tumours derived from APUD cells have been divided into three types for classification purposes: *Type one* have characteristic secretory granules and include oat cell carcinoma of the lung which commonly secretes ACTH, pancreatic islet cell tumour which secrete insulin, gastrin, glucagon and somatostatin and medullary carcinoma of the thyroid associated with calcitonin secretion. *Type two* tumours do not have characteristic secretory granules and are derived from liver, kidney and connective tissue. They secrete hormones like the gonadotrophins and foetal antigens such as alphafetoprotein. *Type three* includes tumours such as phaechromocytomas and neuroblastoma and although they may secrete hormones normally associated with type one tumours such as ACTH, insulin and calcitonin the clinical features associated with type three tumours are most commonly a result of secretion of biogenic amines.

It is easy to recognise, therefore, that development of a hormone producing tumour derived from APUD cells may be associated with a syndrome generally accepted as due to ectopic hormone production, such as ACTH secretion from oat-cell carcinoma of the lung; or such an APUD derived tumour may be associated with a syndrome not related to true ectopic hormone production such as secretion of insulin by a beta-cell tumour of the pancreatic islets.

The APUD concept also helps to explain why multiple endocrine neoplasia occurs and why ectopic tumours may be associated with tumours of endocrine glands in the same patient. For example, gastrin secretion by a pancreatic tumour could be considered to be ectopic but it is frequently found with pituitary tumours and parathyroid tumours in multiple endocrine neoplasia. The cause of multiple hormone producing tumours in this condition is unknown; presumably some defect during development of the neural crest and migration of cells to the various tissue occurs. This defect can be inherited and manifest itself by uncontrolled division of APUD cells leading to multiple hormone producing tumours.

The basic defect that occurs during development is unknown. It has been suggested that it represents de-differentiation and gene derepression without the precise processing and secretory controls found in cells that normally secrete the hormones; this might explain why many endocrine syndromes are associated with production of large amounts of biosynthetic precursors like pro-insulin and 'Big ACTH' rather than the authentic hormone. However, there is evidence that specific gene derepression is not the cause of ectopic hormone production and that failure to control the intracellular abundance of messenger RNA coding for a specific hormone rather than new synthesis from previously inactive genes is responsible [38]. It is possible that hormone synthesis is a universal concomitant of neoplasia but only when the tumours can process biosynthetic precursors to authentic hormones does a clinically recognisable syndrome develop. Clearly this has important implications not only with regard to neoplastic transformation of cells but also to normal cellular differentiation [39].

2.3. Ectopic ACTH syndrome

In a prospective survey of patients with abnormal chest X-ray Wolfson and Odell [40] reported increased levels of a large molecular weight form of ACTH in 72% of patients subsequently shown to have lung cancer. However clinical features ascribed to excessive ACTH secretion occur in as few as 2% of patients with lung cancer [41]. Oat cell tumours of the lung account for 60% of all patients with ectopic ACTH syndrome, thymic tumours 15%, pancreatic tumours 10%, bronchial adenoma 4% and the remaining 11% from a variety of neoplasms [42].

Clinically the syndrome of ectopic production was first defined by Meador *et al.* [43] who demonstrated elevated ACTH activity in plasma and tumours and showed decreased ACTH activity in the pituitaries of five patients with cancer, three of which were bronchogenic in origin. Characteristically, one can expect to find ectopic ACTH syndrome in a middle-aged male who complains of weakness, weight loss, thirst and polyuria, peripheral oedema, perhaps increase in pigmentation, and who will be found subsequently to have glycosuria and probably hypertension. The typical features of Cushings syndrome will rarely be seen except in patients with bronchial carcinoids, thymomas or pancreatic tumours. The patient will have a hypokalaemic alkalosis and abnormal glucose tolerance. Elevated levels of plasma cortisol without diurnal variation will be found and will be resistant to suppression by dexamethasone. Very high levels of immunoassayable ACTH may be detected and in the urine there will be increased excretion of free cortisol, 17 hydroxycorticosteroids and 17 oxosteroids and there will usually be no change with administration of metyrapone.

In one of the five patients described by Meador *et al.* [43] treatment with cytotoxic drugs markedly reduced urinary steroid excretion but the patient died four days after stopping a three day course of treatment. In 1965 Liddle observed that 'with a few salubrious exceptions the treatment of ectopic ACTH syndrome had been unrewarding': in only 3 of 37 patients was surgical removal of the neoplasm followed by apparent cure of the ectopic ACTH syndrome [44]. Seven years later Ratcliffe *et al.* [45] reported falls in plasma ACTH in all five patients who were operated on but one patient died soon after, and in another the relief was only temporary. Unfortunately this dismal picture in ectopic ACTH syndrome remains the rule rather than the exception particularly in patients with lung cancer: In a later study from Liddle's group in only 11 of 105 patients with Cushing's syndrome due to ectopic ACTH production was there an apparent cure following surgical removal of the primary neoplasm [46]. In the evaluation of the use of ACTH measurement as an index of response to treatment of lung cancer Hansen *et al.* found sub-clinical elevation of ACTH in about one-third of their patients [47, 48]. Almost 70% showed a decrease in the hormone level with treatment but this was no help in predicting survival. In general it appears that if a patient has clinical manifestations of ectopic ACTH syndrome, relief of his symptoms by resection of a malignant primary tumour will be exceptional although resection of a more benign tumour like a bronchial carcinoid may be successful [49].

2.4. Inappropriate secretion of antidiuretic hormone (ADH)

Inappropriately increased concentrations of ADH have been reported in 70% of patients with lung cancer but clinical manifestations are rare [47, 48]. The vast majority of cases have been described in patients with oat-cell carcinoma of the lung but there are isolated reports of the syndrome in duodenal and pancreatic cancer [50, 51 ,52]. The clinical syndrome is marked, in extreme cases, by features of water intoxication. These include nausea, vomiting, headache, weakness, lethargy, irritability, confusion, fits and possible coma; the patient may also be oliguric. The biochemical hallmarks of the syndrome are hyponatremia, hypotonic plasma with high urine osmolality, low blood urea and increased concentrations of urinary and plasma ADH. There may also be hypokalaemia and hypocalcaemia [53]. Surgical resection of a tumour can lead to prompt disappearance of the syndrome [54]. Reappearance of the syndrome has been reported with tumour recurrence [55]. Similarly, chemotherapy directed at the primary tumour can be successful in achieving remission of the syndrome, and reduction in levels of ADH have been reported in 60% of patients with lung cancer after treatment of the tumour [56]. But, treatment of the primary tumour is often without effect and in any case reduction in elevated ADH levels is unrelated to survival [47, 48, 57]. Indeed there is some evidence that the presence of the syndrome is, in itself, a poor prognostic feature [47, 48].

2.5. *Zollinger-Ellison syndrome*

Clinical features of Zollinger-Ellison (ZE) syndrome include recalciticant peptic ulcer disease, gastric acid hypersecretion and pancreatic islet cell tumours. The syndrome may account for up to 1% of operative cases of peptic ulcer disease. It occurs most frequently in males between the third and fifth decade of life. Ninety-three percent of patients have peptic ulcer associated with pain as the most prominent symptom. Diarrhoea, vomiting, haematemesis and melaena are all common complaints [58]. Multiple ulcers in duodenum and stomach are common and they may even occur in the jejunum [59]. The diagnosis of ZE syndrome is best made by detecting elevated levels of circulating gastrin before or if necessary after provocative tests [60]. It has been suggested that there are two types of ZE syndrome, one associated with gastric G-cell hyperplasia and another associated with pancreatic gastrinoma. It seems likely, however, that tumours in the pancreas or duodenum account for the vast majority and that G-cell hyperplasia is rare [61, 62]. Two-thirds of the tumours are likely to be malignant and the majority of these will have metastasized by the time the diagnosis has been established. Total gastrectomy is the treatment of choice with resection of the pancreatic tumour if possible. Successful treatment (by total gastrectomy and pancreatic tumour resection) will be associated with relief of symptoms and a fall in serum gastrin but persistent elevation of serum gastrin does not appear to have prognostic significance [60]. It should be remembered that ZE syndrome commonly occurs with multiple endocrine neoplasia (see below) and the glands most frequently involved are the pituitary and the parathyroids. Furthermore, this syndrome is familial so that it may be wise to screen and follow up close relatives [63].

2.6. *Calcitonin and medullary carcinoma of the thyroid and ectopic calcitonin production*

Medullary carcinoma of the thyroid, a calcitonin secreting tumour, is rare and accounts for only about 9% of all patients with thyroid cancer [64]. The male/female incidence in this condition is 1.4:1 compared with 2.5:1 in other types of thyroid cancer. The age range at diagnosis in the series by Hill [64] was 15–82 with an average of 47. Up to 50% of patients have disease not localised to the thyroid at the time of diagnosis and unfortunately there are often no symptoms until a thyroid nodule is noticed in the neck by the patient. Presentation because of a metastatic nodule is also common. Diarrhoea occurs in up to one-third of patients and is frequently associated with extensive disease. The tumours when palpable are hard and often very tender to palpation. Metastases occur frequently in cervical lymph nodes and sometimes in liver. Medullary carcinoma of the thyroid may be sporadic or familial and it may be associated with parathyroid tumours and with phaeochromocytoma in multiple endocrine neoplasia. Several large kindreds with this type of multiple endocrine neoplasia have been studied. Serum calcitonin levels are markedly raised in patients with medullary carcinoma of the thyroid [65, 66, 67]. Hypocalcaemia, however, is rare; paradoxically in the presence of a parathyroid tumour, hypercalcaemia may be present. Measurement of serum calcitonin either basally or stimulated (see below) is of definite value in the diagnosis of medullary carcinoma in patients with thyroid nodules. Moreover, in familial medullary carcinoma of the thyroid and in relatives of patients with multiple endocrine neoplasia, elevation of serum calcitonin can lead to early diagnosis in apparently unaffected members of a kindred even before thyroid nodules appear.

2.6.1. The use of calcitonin measurements as an index of tumour response to treatment. Detection of increased levels of calcitonin by radioimmunoassay is an effective screening method for early diagnosis of occult disease as well as for patients with thyroid nodules. It is also of considerable help in detecting persistent or recurrent medullary carcinoma of the thyroid following surgery. The usefulness of calcitonin measurement as a tumour marker is further enhanced by stimulatory tests using agents such as calcium and/or pentagastrin [68]. Intravenous administration of calcium and pentagastrin together appears to be the most useful screening test for occult primary or metastatic medullary carcinoma of the thyroid. Patients who are relatives of affected members of a kindred in whom the diagnosis is made on the basis of calcitonin measurements, particularly following provocative testing, have less extensive disease than those who present with thyroid nodules [68].

Following surgery (usually total thyroidectomy $\pm$ lymph node dissection) the serum calcitonin level falls and in successfully treated early cases may become undetectable. In a proportion of patients persistent elevation of serum calcitonin can be found without clinical evidence of residual tumour. Further neck operations may not be successful in reducing calcitonin levels even if further medullary carcinoma is found and removed. This suggests that microscopic metastases are present which may remain dormant for many years and are detectable only because of the sensitivity of the biochemical test. However, progressively increasing levels of hormone indicate extension of the disease [67].

The disease can be cured, as evidenced by the fact that 11 of 72 patients described by Hill *et al.* [64] were still alive 10 years after initial treatment. However, in the same series 15 patients rapidly went downhill and had a mean survival of only 22 months. A third group had an average period of remission of 81 months, then tumour recurrence or metastases developed and the average total survival from initial treatment was 107 months. Because of the high incidence of recurrence even after apparent cure, periodic re-evaluation with calcitonin measurements (after provocative tests if necessary) will allow early detection of functioning neoplastic tissue.

2.6.2. Calcitonin secretion by other tumours. Very high levels of calcitonin in serum are seen only in medullary carcinoma of the thyroid. However, there is now a great deal of evidence that other cancers can be associated with hypercalcitoninaemia. Silva *et al.* [69] first reported the case of a 65-year-old male with an oat-cell carcinoma of the lung who had markedly elevated concentrations of calcitonin that declined with treatment. Moreover, catheterisation of a vein draining the tumour revealed a very high level of hormone compared with that in the blood from the inferior thyroid vein draining the thyroid. Subsequently Milhaud and his colleagues [70] described their experience over the preceding 6-year period in which they had found elevated serum calcitonin levels in patients with a wide variety of cancers derived from the neural crest. In the same year Coombes *et al.* [71] reported increased concentrations of calcitonin in plasma samples from 21 of 46 patients with non-thyroid cancer and that the concentration of the hormone could be increased during calcium infusion. In addition, they suggested that serial estimations of calcitonin in plasma might be useful in assessing the response of non-thyroid tumours to treatment; this was substantiated in four patients described by Mulder and Hackeng [72] in whom serum calcitonin following treatment was lower than before treatment. In a blind prospective survey of 100 patients with a variety of cancers Schwartz *et al.* [73] found elevated levels of calcitonin in 38% of patients with cancer of the lung, 24% with cancer of the colon, 38% with cancer of the breast, 42% with cancer of the pancreas and 30% with gastric carcinoma. Unfortunately, in these patients, however, post treatment values were little different from those obtained before treatment. In only one patient with a successfully treated colonic cancer did serum calcitonin fall to normal and this was found to be elevated again one month before a malignant colonic polyp was found.

Schwartz *et al.* commented that this might be a reflection of the generally unsatisfactory treatment for these tumours; moreover, the frequency of hypercalcitoninaemia, particularly in the common cancers of the lung and breast, tends to be higher in those patients with skeletal metastases for whom there is often little to offer apart from palliative treatment. However, Silva *et al.* [74], having found hypercalcitoninaemia in 58% of 61 patients with bronchogenic cancer, suggested that it might be a useful marker to assess treatment of cancer since anti-tumour therapy caused a significant decrease in calcitonin levels in 75% of patients after treatment.

2.7. *Tumour hypoglycaemia*

The most well-recognised but nevertheless rare cause of hypoglycaemia due to a hormone secreting tumour is the islet cell tumour or insulinoma. The great majority of these are benign adenomas which are small and evenly distributed throughout the pancreas. Only rarely are they found in ectopic sites, usually along the gastrointestinal tract. Some extra-pancreatic tumours can cause hypoglycaemia, the majority of these being large mesenchymal tumours or tumours of the liver. Extra-pancreatic tumours do not usually secrete insulin and the cause of hypoglycaemia in these cases has not yet been established but 'non-suppressible insulin-like activity' which may be related to somatomedins is one of the factors that has been incriminated [75]. Whatever the cause of tumour hypoglycaemia the presenting features are similar. Of some importance is the fact that symptoms may be bizarre and the diagnosis unsuspected for several years. Uncharacteristic behaviour patterns, confusional states and disturbances of consciousness are the most common features. Hunger is unusual and there may not be the increase in weight that one might expect with chronic hypoglycaemia. Whatever the symptoms they are exacerbated by fasting, occur often in the early morning and are alleviated by eating.

Differentiation between insulinoma and extrapancreatic hypoglycaemia is usually not difficult. Patients with insulinoma have inappropriately high concentrations of insulin or pro-insulin in the presence of a low blood sugar. Patients with extrapancreatic tumours have low insulin levels. A number of tests have been described using assays of insulin, pro-insulin or C-peptide which help to establish the diagnosis of insulinoma [76]. Pre-operative localisation of a tumour helps identification at operation and reduces the risk of missing the insulinoma which will occur in 75% of patients if a blind distal pancreatectomy is performed [77]. Successful removal of an insulinoma will result in remission of symptoms and a fall in insulin levels.

2.8. *Ectopic pituitary hormones other than ACTH and ADH*

2.8.1. Growth hormone (GH) and prolactin. Ectopic production of GH is not well documented, primarily because GH is a stress hormone and any elevation in serum in association with cancer may be coincidental. However, Steiner *et al.* [78] demonstrated a fall in immunoreactive GH in one patient, who had lung cancer associated with osteoarthropathy, after resection of his tumour; moreover, post-operatively his knee and ankle pains disappeared. Similarly Greenberg *et al.* [79] described a patient whose hypertrophic pulmonary osteoarthropathy disappeared following resection of a lung tumour shown to synthesize GH *in vitro*. However, the association between ectopic GH secretion and osteoarthropathy is inconsistent so that the clinical responses to therapy are not necessarily related.

There have been few reports of non-pituitary tumours secreting prolactin. Turkington [80] described two patients with hyperprolactinaemia – one a male with an undifferentiated bronchogenic neoplasm, the other female with a hypernephroma. In the first patient there were no symptoms attributable to hyperprolactinaemia but in the female with a hypernephroma there was a short history of galactorrhoea. In both patients prolactin levels fell following treatment of the primary tumour, the lung cancer by radiotherapy and the hypernephroma by surgical resection. Rees *et al.* [81] reported that prolactin was one of a wide variety of hormones secreted by an oat-cell carcinoma of the lung. Initially it seemed likely that ectopic hyperprolactinaemia would be relatively unusual since none of 20 patients screened by Turkington [80] had any increase in serum prolactin levels. This was substantiated by the fact that in a series of over 100 patients in whom elevation of at least one hormone such as ACTH or calcitonin was found in up to 80% of cases, elevated prolactin levels were found in only two cases [41].

2.8.2. Gonadotrophins [39, 82]. As already mentioned in the introduction to this section human chorionic gonadotrophins are well established as markers of chorioncarcinoma and are discussed in detail elsewhere in this book (Chapter 3). Elevated levels of gonadotrophins are also found in blood and urine of patients who have other tumours of trophoblastic origin, e.g. teratocarcinoma of testis and ovary. Strictly speaking gonadotrophin production by these tumours is not ectopic. However, the clinical association between precocious puberty, gynaecomastia and malignant disease is well recognised and has been reported in a variety of tumours of non-trophoblastic origin including carcinoma of the lung and liver [83]. In fact Odell and Wolfsen [82] have produced evidence that gonadotrophins are frequently elevated in patients with cancer but that they produce few or no symptoms. It should be emphasised that gynaecomastia is frequently found in adults with cancer and is probably more likely to be due to concomitant liver disease or drug administration than to excessive ectopic gonadotrophin production.

2.8.3. Thyrotrophin (TSH). Trophoblastic tumours can be associated with mild hyperthyroidism and the tumour hormone responsible has been shown to have TSH-like biological activity but little immuno-reactivity. There is some suggestion that this hormone, which has been called human chorionic thyrotrophin, is in fact human chorionic gonadotrophin. Hyperthyroidism is usually mild but there have been reports of severe symptoms that remitted following resection of tumour [84].

2.9. *Placental hormones*

2.9.1. Human chorionic gonadotrophin. This hormone is considered in detail in Chapter 3.

2.9.2. Human placental lactogen (HPL). Ectopic production of HPL by tissues other than those derived from placenta or trophoblast was described by Fusco and Rosen [85] in a male with bronchogenic carcinoma. Subsequently a report appeared of increased concentrations of HPL in the serum of a male with gynaecomastia associated with carcinoma of the lung [86]. Weintraub and Rosen [87] found detectable HPL in 11 of 128 patients with various malignancies other than those originating from trophoblast or gonad. The presence of HPL is not necessarily associated with any clinical features but some patients have had gynaecomastia [88].

2.10. *Gastrointestinal hormones*

2.10.1. Glucagon [89, 90, 91]. A rare syndrome associated with hypersecretion of glucagon has been described in which the patients (who are usually female, between the ages of 48 and 65 but occasionally younger) present with a skin rash (known as necrolytic migratory erythema), glossitis, weight loss and symptoms of diabetes mellitus. The patients have very high levels of glucagon in their plasma and have tumours (usually malignant) of the alpha cells of the pancreas. Resection of the tumour has been reported to result in prompt remission of all symptoms with rapid normalisation of plasma glucagon. A syndrome caused by ectopic secretion of enteroglucagon (now known as glicentin) has also been described in which a renal tumour was associated with constipation, oedema, hair loss, amenorrhoea and a transient skin rash, all of which resolved following removal of the involved kidney [92, 93].

2.10.2. Vaso-active intestinal peptide (VIP) [91, 94]. Watery diarrhoea (sustained or intermittent) with hypokalaemia, hypochlorhydria and less frequently hyperglycaemia and hypercalcaemia have been recognised as a humoral syndrome (Verner-Morrison syndrome) associated mainly with pancreatic tumours but also with bronchogenic cancer. The pancreatic tumours may be benign or malignant and the evidence supports the suggestion that hypersecretion of VIP by these tumours is responsible for the symptoms. Surgical resection of adenomas or medical treatment with steroids or streptozotocin can not only alleviate symptoms and correct the biochemical abnormalities but also result in a fall in plasma VIP levels.

2.10.3. Other hormones. Excessive somatostatin secretion from a pancreatic tumour may cause diabetes, steatorrhoea and gallstones. Resection of the tumour has been followed by complete remission of symptoms [95, 96]. Pancreatic polypeptide, though not obviously responsible for a specific syndrome, has been reported to be elevated in two-thirds of patients with Verner-Morrison syndrome, half of patients with glucagonomas and a quarter of patients with gastrinomas or insulinomas. Thus it may be a useful diagnostic aid for detection of pancreatic tumours.

2.11. The carcinoid syndrome [97]

Carcinoid tumours are derived from enterochromaffin cells which are part of the APUD cell series originating in the neural crest. Tumours can be classified as arising from embryonic foregut, midgut or hindgut. Embryonic foregut tumours are found in the lung, pancreas and stomach, midgut tumours in the ileum and hindgut tumours in the rectum and colon. The carcinoid syndrome has also been described in associated with tumours of the ovary, cervix uteri and testis. As well as secreting 5HT, kallikrein, histamine and prostaglandins, carcinoids may secrete a variety of hormones including ACTH, insulin, motilin and VIP.

Clinically patients commonly present with facial flushing and swelling, lacrimation, diarrhoea and abdominal discomfort, asthma and congestive cardiac failure (due to cardiac lesions including pulmonary valvular stenosis). Some bronchial carcinoids are not associated with the characteristic syndrome; they may secrete predominantly ACTH which can cause Cushing's syndrome indistinguishable from that due to a pituitary adenoma or they may secrete insulin and be associated with hypoglycaemia. Tumour resection can lead to cure of carcinoid syndrome (or Cushing's syndrome if ACTH is secreted); however, a proportion of carcinoid tumours are malignant and metastases preclude surgical treatment.

2.12. Multiple endocrine neoplasia

Multiple endocrine adenomatosis or neoplasia is an inherited condition in which patients have tumours of a variety of endocrine glands which manifest themselves as endocrine syndromes. There are at least two distinct types of multiple endocrine neoplasia (MEN). In MEN type I the glands involved in descending order of frequency are the parathyroids, the pituitary and the endocrine pancreas; occasionally the adrenal cortex may be involved [98]. In MEN type II there is involvement of the parathyroids, thyroid (medullary carcinoma) and adrenal medulla (phaeochromocytoma) [99]. A third type where there is a 'marfanoid' habitus and multiple mucosal neuromas with medullary thyroid carcinoma and phaeochromocytoma has also been described [100]. In type I peptic ulceration is a common presenting complaint. Zollinger-Ellison syndrome may occur in up to 40% of patients and elevated serum gastrin levels will establish the diagnosis. In addition, hypercalcaemia due to single or multiple parathyroid tumours may occur and be substantiated by a high circulating immunoassayable parathyroid hormone concentrations. In up to 65% of patients a pituitary adenoma will be found; this was thought to be non-functioning in the majority of cases but recent evidence suggests that many of these patients have hyperprolactinaemia which may or may not be associated with galactorrhoea and amenorrhoea in females [101]. An additional feature of this syndrome is the occurrence of bronchial carcinoids which seem only rarely to cause any endocrine disturbance, although high circulating levels of serotonin may be found. In MEN Type II, familial phaeochromocytoma with medullary carcinoma of the thyroid is the most frequent combination. In an analysis of 85 reported cases of familial phaeochromocytoma [99] 14 also had medullary carcinoma of the thyroid. Parathyroid tumours have been reported in association with familial phaeochromocytoma and the combination of all three was found in 5 of the 85 reported cases reviewed by Steiner *et al.* [99]. In so-called MEN Type III 38 of 41 patients had medullary carcinoma of the thyroid, 19 had phaeochromocytoma and all of them had some sort of soft tissue defect such as neuroma, 'marfanoid' habitus or gastrointestinal abnormalities [100].

In these syndromes resection of the appropriate endocrine tumour is followed by correction of the biochemical abnormality and alleviation of the symptoms. It is important to remember that these conditions are inherited and there is some evidence of shared HLA haplotype [101]; it is therefore important to screen near relatives by the appropriate biochemical or hormonal measurement and this is particularly true of children since the disorder may not manifest itself until the second decade of life.

3. Summary

Hypercalcaemia in cancer is common and is mainly associated with bony metastases. Only in a relatively small group of patients who have solid tumours without bony metastases is correction of hypercalcaemia consistently useful as an index of tumour response to treatment. In patients with an ACTH syndrome usually due to carcinoma of the bronchus, levels of circulating hormones do not often fall following treatment of the primary tumour and in any case such a fall is unrelated to survival; therefore hormone measurement in this situation is not helpful as a reliable index of successful treatment. Only in the occasional patient with a bronchial carcinoid associated with ACTH production is a fall in circulating hormone concentration a good indicator of successful treatment. In the syndrome of inappropriate secretion of ADH a fall in immunoassayable ADH often occurs following treatment of the primary tumour but such a fall is unrelated to survival.

In medullary carcinoma of the thyroid assay of calcitonin cannot only be successful in predicting tumour response to treatment but also in indicating tumour recurrence. Moreover, measurement of serum calcitonin in apparently unaffected relatives of patients with familial disease may allow detection of occult tumour. In patients with non-thyroid tumours secreting calcitonin, changes in immunoassayable hormone levels are unhelpful and in any case prognosis in this group is usually poor.

In tumours of the gastrointestinal tract hormone measurements are sometimes useful in indicating successful treatment, for example in insulinoma, Zollinger-Ellison syndrome (if the tumour can be found and removed), Verner-Morrison (excessive VIP) syndrome, glucagonoma and the very rare somatostatinoma. Similarly, successful treatment of benign carcinoid tumour can be followed by alleviation of the associated endocrine syndrome and a fall in hormone level. Tumours that secrete pituitary and placental-like hormones other than chorioncarcinoma (considered elsewhere) are rare and hormone measurements may or may not be helpful in providing information about successful treatment.

In multiple endocrine neoplasia, hormone measurements may allow early detection of parathyroid, pituitary, pancreatic, adrenal and thyroid (medullary carcinoma) tumours. Successful removal of the tumour is followed by correction of the endocrine syndrome and a fall in circulating hormone concentration. Furthermore, screening of apparently unaffected relatives particularly with serum calcium and calcitonin estimations might result in early detection of the syndrome.

References

1. Myers WPL: Hypercalcaemia in neoplastic disease. Arch Surg 80:308–318, 1960.
2. Galasko CS, Burns JI: Hypercalcaemia in patients with advanced mammary cancer. Br Med J 3:573–577, 1971.
3. Paterson JS, Baum M: Safety of tamoxifen. Lancet i:105, 1978.
4. Mundy GR, Eilon G, Orr W, Spiro TP, Yoneda T: Osteoclast activating factor: its role in myeloma and other types of hypercalcaemia of malignancy. Metabolic Bone Disease and Related Research 2:173–176, 1980.
5. Powles TJ, Clarke SA, Easty DM, Easty GE, Munro-Neville A: The inhibition by aspirin and indomethacin of osteolytic tumour deposits and hypercalcaemia in rats with Walker tumour and its possible applications to human breast cancer. Br J Cancer 28:316–321, 1973.

6. Powles TJ, Dowsett M, East GC, Easty DM, Munro-Neville A: Breast cancer, osteolysis, bone metastasis and anti-osteolytic effect of aspirin. Lancet i:608–610, 1976.
7. Coomes RC, Munro-Neville A, Bondy PK *et al.*: Failure of indomethacin to reduce hypercalcaemia in patients with breast cancer. Prostaglandins 12(6):1027–1035, 1976.
8. Richmond J, Sherman RS, Diamond HD, Craver LF: Renal lesions associated with malignant lymphomas. Am J Med 32:184–207, 1962.
9. Canellos GP: Hypercalcaemia in malignant lymphoma and leukaemia. Ann NY Acad Sci 230:240–246, 1974.
10. Greaves M, Hancock BW: Hypercalcaemia in malignant lymphoma. Postgrad Med J 56 (651):34–37.
11. Mundy GR, Rick ME, Turcotte R, Kowalski MA: Pathogenesis of hypercalcaemia in lymphocarcoma cell leukaemia – role of an osteoclast activating factor-like substance and a mechanism of action for glucocorticoid therapy. Am J Med 65:600–606, 1978.
12. Horton JE, Raisz LG, Simmon HA, Oppenheim JJ, Mergenhagen SE: Bone resorbing activity in supernatant fluid from cultured human peripheral blood leucocytes. Science 177:793–795, 1972.
13. Buckle RM: Ectopic PTH syndrome, pseudohyperparathyroidism hypercalcaemia of malignancy. Clin Endocrinol 3:237–251, 1974.
14. Melick RA, Martin TJ, Hicks JD: Parathyroid hormone production and malignancy. Br Med J (ii):204–205, 1972.
15. Heath DA: Hypercalcaemia and malignancy. Ann Clin Biochem 13:555–560, 1976.
16. Skrabanek P, McPartlin J, Powell D: Tumour hypercalcaemia. Medicine 59:41, 262–282, 1980.
17. Demers LM, Allegra JC, Harvey HA, Lipton H, Luderer JR, Mostel R, Brenner DE: Plasma prostaglandins in hypercalcaemic patients with malignant disease. Cancer 39:1559–1562, 1977.
18. Tashjian AH Jr, Voelkel EF, Levine L, Goldhaber P: Evidence that the bone resorption – stimulating factor produced by mouse fibrosarcoma cells is prostaglandin E2: a new model for the hypercalcaemia of cancer. J Exp Med 136:1329–1342, 1972.
19. Brereton HD, Halushka PV, Alexander RW, Mason DM, Keiser HR, DeVita VT Jr.: Indomethacin responsive hypercalcaemia in a patient with renal-cell adenocarcinoma. N Eng J Med 291:83–85, 1974.
20. Robertson RP, Baylink D.: Elevated prostaglandin E1, hypercalcaemia and suppressed parathyroid hormone in neoplasia in man. Clin Res 23:113a, 1975.
21. Seyberth HW, Segre GV, Morgan JL, Sweetman BJ, Potts JT, Jr. Oates JA: Prostaglandins as mediators of hypercalcaemia associated with certain types of cancer. N Eng J Med 136:1329–1342, 1975.
22. Kennedy BJ, Emerson WJ, Tibbets DM, Nathanson IT, Aub JL: Hypercalcaemia complication of hormone therapy of advanced breast cancer. Cancer Res 13:445–449.
23. Cole MP, Jones CTA, Todd IDH: A new anti-oestrogenic agent in late breast cancer. An early clinical appraisal of ICI 46474. Br J Cancer 25:270–275, 1971.
24. Ward HWC: Antioestrogen therapy for breast cancer; a trial of tamoxifen at 2 dose levels. Br Med J 1:13–14, 1973.
25. Manni A, Trujillo J, Marshall JS, Pearson OH: Antioestrogen-induced remission in stage four breast cancer. Cancer Treat Reports 60:1445–1450, 1976.
26. Kiang DT, Kennedy BJ: Tamoxifen (antioestrogen) therapy in advanced breast cancer. Ann Intern Med 87 (6):687–690, 1977.
27. Veldhuis JD: Tamoxifen and hypercalcaemia. Ann Intern Med 88(4):574–575, 1978.
28. Minton MJ, Cantwell BN, Knight RK, Ruben ED, Hayward JL: Safety of tamofixen. Lancet i:346–397, 1978.
29. Spooner D, Evans BD: Tamoxifen and life threatening hypercalcaemia. Lancet ii:413–414, 1979.

30. Minton MJ, Sparrow G, Rubens RD, Hayward JL: Tamoxifen induced hypercalcaemia and response to treatment. Br Med J 280:186–187, 1980.
31. Coombes RC, Dady P, Parsons C, Powles TJ: Mithromycin therapy, an adjunct to conventional treatment of hypercalcaemia and bone metastasis in breast cancer. Metabolic Bone Disease and Related Research 2:199–202, 1980.
32. Muggia FM, Heineman HO: Hypercalcaemia associated with neoplastic disease. Ann Intern Med 73:281–290, 1970.
33. Lokich J, Shevitz F: Hypercalcaemia in malignant lymphoma, a case in a patient after parathyroidectomy. JAMA 242 (1):66–67, 1979.
34. McArthur JR, Athens JW, Wintrobe MN, Cartwright GE: Melphalan and myeloma: experience with a low-dose continuous regimen. Ann Intern Med 72:665–670, 1970.
35. Powell D, Singer FR, Murray TM, Minkin C, Potts JT Jr.: Non-parathyroid humoral hypercalcaemia in patients with neoplastic disease. N Engl J Med 289:176–181, 1973.
36. Tomlinson S: Investigation of hypercalcaemia. Metabolic Bone Disease and Related Research 3:161–166, 1980.
37. Drezner MK, Lebovitz HE: Primary hyperparathyroidism in paraneoplastic hypercalcaemia. Lancet i (8072):1004–1006, 1978.
38. Shields R: Ectopic hormone production by tumours. Nature 272 (5653):494, 1978.
39. Odell WD, Wolfsen AR: Hormones from tumours; are they ubiquitous? Am J Med 68 (3):317–318, 1980.
40. Wolfsen AR, Odell WD: Pro-ACTH; used for early detection of lung cancer. Am J Med 66 (5):765–772, 1979.
41. Gropp C, Havemann K, Scheuer A: Ectopic hormones in lung cancer patients at diagnosis and during therapy. Cancer 46 (1):347–354, 1980.
42. Amatruda TT, Upton GV: Hyperadrenocorticsm and ACTH releasing factor. Ann NY Acad Sci 230:168, 1974.
43. Meador CK, Liddle GW, Island DP, Nicholson WE, Lucas CP, Nuckton JG, Leutscher JA: Cause of Cushing's syndrome in patients with tumours arising from non-endocrine tissue. J Clin Endocrinol 22:693–703, 1962.
44. Liddle GW, Givens JR, Nicholson WE: The ectopic ACTH syndrome. Cancer Res 25:1057–1061, 1965.
45. Ratcliffe JG, Knight RA, Besser GM, Landon J, Stansfield AG: Tumour and plasma ACTH concentrations in patients with and without ectopic ACTH syndrome. Clin Endocrinol 1:22–44, 1972.
46. Orth DM, Liddle GW: Results of treatment in 108 patients with Cushing's syndrome. N Engl J Med 285:243–247, 1971.
47. Hansen M, Hammer M, Hummer L: ACTH, ADH and calcitonin as markers of response and relapse in small cell carcinoma of the lung. Cancer 46 (2):2062–2067.
48. Hansen M, Hammer M, Hummer L: Diagnostic and therapeutic implications of ectopic hormone production in small cell carcinoma of the lung. Thorax 35 (2):101–105, 1980.
49. Vingerhoeds ACM, der Kinderen PJ, Thijssen JHH, Schwarz F: Detection of an ACTH-secreting bronchial carcinoid tumour 18 months after adrenalectomy for Cushing's syndrome. Acta Endocrinol 67:625–633, 1971.
50. Marks LJ, Berde B, Klein LA, Roth J, Goonan SR, Blumen D, Nabseth DC: Inappropriate vasopressin secretion and carcinoma of the pancreas. Am J Med 45:967–974, 1968.
51. Lebacq E, Delaere J: Origine des substances antidiuretiques et explication de l'hypernatriurie dans le syndrome de Schwartz Bartter. Annales D'Endocrinologie 26:375, 1965.
52. Vorherr H, Massry S, Utiger RD, Kleeman CR: Antidiuretic principle in malignant tumour extract from patients with inappropriate ADH syndrome. J Clin Endocrinol Metab 28:162–168, 1968.
53. De Troyer A, Demanet JC: Clinical, biochemical and pathogenic features of the syndrome

of inappropriate secretion of antidiuretic hormones. A review of 26 cases with marked hyponatraemia. Quart J Med 45:180, 521–531, 1976.
54. Utiger RD: Inappropriate anti-diuresis and carcinoma of the lung. Detection of arginine vasopressin in tumour extracts by immunoassay. J Clin Endocrinol Metab 26:970–974, 1966.
55. Tisher CL: Correction of an ADH syndrome by resection of a bronchogenic carcinoma with demonstration of tumour antidiuretic activity. Clin Res 14:185, 1966.
56. Linton AL, Hutton I: Hyponatremia and bronchial carcinoma. Therapy with nitrogen mustard. Br Med J 2: 277–278, 1965.
57. Bartter ST, Schwartz WB: The syndrome of inappropriate secretion of antidiuretic hormone. Am J Med 42:790–806, 1967.
58. Ellison EH, Wilson GD: The Zollinger Ellison syndrome: reappraisal and evaluation of 260 registered cases. Ann Surg 160:512–530, 1964.
59. Hallenbeck: The Zollinger-Ellison syndrome. Gastroenterol 54:426–422, 1968.
60. Deveney CW, Deveney KS, Way LW: The Zollinger-Ellison syndrome – 23 years later. Ann Surg 188 (3):384–393, 1978.
61. Polak JM, Stagg B, Pearse AGE: Two types of Zollinger-Ellison syndrome: immunofluorescence, cytochemical and ultrastructural studies of the antral pancreatic gastrin cells in different clinical states. Gut 13:501–512, 1972.
62. Fox PS, Hofmann JW, Wilson SD, De Coss JJ: Surgical management of the Zollinger-Ellison syndrome. Surg Clin North Am 54:395–407, 1974.
63. Tomlinson S: Multiple endocrine adenomatosis and peptic ulcer. Proc R Soc Med 66:445–446, 1973.
64. Hill CS, Ibanez NL, Samaan NA, Ahearn MJ, Clark RL: Medullary (solid) carcinoma of the thyroid gland: an analysis of the MD Anderson hospital experience with patients with the tumour, its special features and its histogenesis. Medicine 52:141–171, 1973.
65. Tashjian AH, Melvin KEW: Medullary carcinoma of the thyroid gland: studies of thyrocalcitonin in plasma and tumour extracts. N Engl J Med 279:279–283, 1968.
66. Tubiana M, Millhaud G, Courtris D, Lacour J, Parmentier C, Bok B: Medullary carcinoma and thyrocalcitonin. Br Med J 4:87–89, 1968.
67. Block MA, Jackson CE, Tashjian AH: Management of occult medullary thyroid carcinoma evidenced only by serum calcitonin level elevations after apparently adequate neck operations. Arch Surg 113 (4):368–372, 1978.
68. Wells SA, Baylin SB, Linehan WM, Farrell RE, Cocks EB, Cooper CW: Provocative agents and the diagnosis of medullary carcinoma of thyroid gland. Ann Surg 188 (2):139–141, 1978.
69. Silva OL, Becher KL, Primack A, Doppman J, Snider RH: Ectopic secretion of calcitonin by oat-cell carcinoma. N Eng J Med 290:1122–1124, 1974.
70. Milhaud G, Calmette C, Taboulet J, Julienne A, Moukhtar MS: Hypersecretion of calcitonin in neoplastic conditions. Lancet i:462–463, 1974.
71. Coombes RC, Hillyard C, Greenberg PB, McIntyre I: Plasma immunoreactive clacitonin in patients with non-thyroid tumours. Lancet i:1080–1083, 1974.
72. Mulder H, Hackeng WHL: Ectopic secretion of calcitonin. Acta Med Scand 204 (4):253–256, 1978.
73. Schwartz KE, Wolfsen AR, Forster B, Odell WD: Calcitonin in non-thyroidal cancer. J Clin Endocrinol Metab 49:438–444, 1979.
74. Silva OL, Broder LE, Doppman JL, Snider RA, Moore CF, Cohen MH, Becker KL: Calcitonin as a marker for bronchogenic cancer. A prospective study. Cancer 44:680–684, 1979.
75. Megyesi K, Kahn CR, Roth J, Gorden P: Circulating NSILA-s in man: preliminary studies of stimuli in vivo and binding to plasma components. J Clin Endocrinol Metab 41:475–484, 1975.

76. Editorial: Diagnosis and treatment of insulin secreting tumours. Lancet i:22–23, 1980.
77. Mengoli L, LeQuesne LP: Blind pancreatic resection for suspected insulinoma: a review of the problem. Br J Surg 54:749–756, 1967.
78. Steiner H, Dahlback O, Waldenstarm J: Ectopic growth hormone production and osteoarthropathy in carcinoma of the bronchus. Lancet i:783–785, 1968.
79. Greenberg PB, Beck C, Martin TJ, Burger HG: Synthesis and release of human growth hormone from lung carcinoma in cell culture. Lancet i:350–352, 1972.
80. Turkington RW: Ectopic production of prolactin. N Eng J Med 285:1455–1458, 1971.
81. Rees LH, Bloomfield GA, Rees GM, Corin B, Franks LN, Ratcliffe JG: Multiple hormones in a bronchial tumour. J Clin Endocrinol Metab 38:1090–1097, 1974.
82. Odell WD, Wolfsen AR: Humoral syndromes associated with cancer. Annu Rev Med 29:379–406, 1978.
83. Rees LH, Ratcliffe JG: Ectopic hormone production by non-endocrine tumours. Clin Endocrinol 3:263–299, 1974.
84. Hershmann JN, Higgins HP, Starnes WR: Differences between thyroid stimulator in hydatidifotmmole and human chorionic thyrotrophin. Metabolism 19:735–740, 1970.
85. Fusco FD, Rosen SW: Gonadotrophin producing anaplastic large-cell carcinoma of the lung. N Eng J Med 275:507–515, 1966.
86. Grumbach NN, Kaplan S, Sciarra JJ, Burr IN: Chorionic growth hormone - prolactin (CGP): secretion, disposition, and biologic activity in man, and postulated function as the growth hormone of the second half of pregnancy. Ann NY Acad Sci 148:501–531, 1968.
87. Weintraub BC, Rosen S: Ectopic production of human chorionic somatotrophin by non-trophoblastic cancers. J Clin Endocrinol Metab 32:94–101, 1971.
88. Blackman NR, Rosen SW, Weintraub BC: Ectopic hormones. Adv Intern Med 23:85–113, 1978.
89. Mallinson CN, Bloom SR, Warin AD, Salmon PR, Cox B: A glucagonona syndrome. Lancet ii:1–5, 1974.
90. Swenson KH, Amon RD, Hanifin JN: The glucagonoma syndrome a distinctive cutaneous marker of systemic disease. Arch Dermatol 114:224–228, 1978.
91. Bloom SR, Polak JN: Gut hormones. Adv Clin Chem 21:177–244, 1980.
92. Gleeson NH, Bloom SR, Polak JN, Henry K, Dowling RH: Endocrine tumour in kidney effecting small bowel structure and absorptive function. Gut 12:773–782, 1971.
93. Bloom SR: An enteroglucagon tumour. Gut 13:520–523, 1972.
94. Said S., Faloona GR: Elevated plasma and tissue levels of vasoactive intestinal polypeptide in the Watery-diarrhoea syndrome due to pancreatic, bronchogenic and other tumours. N Engl J Med 293:155–160, 1975.
95. Larsson LI, Hirsch MA, Holst JJ, Ingemansson S, Kuhl C, Lindkaer Jensen S, Lundqvist G, Rehfeld JF, Schwartz TW: Pancreatic somatostatinoma clinical features and physiological implications. Lancet i:666–668, 1977.
96. Ganda OP, Weir GC, Soeldner JS, Legg MA, Chick WL, Patel YC, Ebeid AM, Gabbay KH, Reichlin S: Somatostatinoma, a somatostatin containing tumour of the endocrine pancreas. N Eng J Med 296 (17):963–967, 1977.
97. Graham-Smith DG: The carcinoid syndrome, pp 1721–1731. In: Endocrinology, vol. 3, DeGroot LJ, Gahil GF, Odell WD, Martini L, Potts JT Jr, Nelson DH, Steinberger E, Winegrad AI (eds). Grune and Streatton, 1979.
98. Ballard HS, Frame B, Hartsock RJ: Multiple endocrine adenoma and peptic ulcer complex. Medicine 43:481–516, 1964.
99. Steiner AL, Goodman AD, Powers SR: Studies of a kindred with phaechromocytoma, medullary thyroid carcinoma, hyperparathyroidism, and Cushing's disease: multiple endocrine neoplasia type 2. Medicine 47:371–409, 1968.

100. Khairi MR, Dexter RN, Burzynski NJ, Johnston CC: Mucosal neuroma, phaeochromocytoma and medullary thyroid carcinoma; multiple endocrine neoplasia type 3. Medicine 54:89–112, 1975.
101. Farid NR, Buehler S, Russell NA, Maroun FB, Allerdice P, Smyth HS: Prolactinomas in familial multiple endocrine neoplasia syndrome type 1, relationship to HLA and carcinoid tumours. Am J Med 69:874–880, 1980.

6. Haematological Changes

B. W. HANCOCK and J. RICHMOND

1. Introduction

In the follow-up of patients with cancer, haematological disturbances are many and varied. They may affect the formed elements, immune function, coagulation and the erythrocyte sedimentation rate. There may be special effects from splenic involvement in the disease and from splenectomy. In addition, striking abnormalities of iron, vitamin B12 and folate metabolism can occur.

2. Red cell abnormalities

2.1. *Anaemia*

Anaemia is very common in patients with malignant disease at some stage of their illness; it is more often a feature of widespread or recurrent tumour than of localised responding disease and as such may be regarded as a good marker of tumour status. Simple investigations after pertinent history and examination will often reveal the cause (see Table 1).

2.1.1. Deficiency anaemias are sometimes multifactorial but isolated deficiencies of iron, from chronic haemorrhage or inadequate diet, of folic acid and less often of vitamin B12, may be seen (see section 8). Megaloblastic features in the marrow are sometimes found in the absence of folic acid or B12 deficiency in patients with malignant disease; cytotoxic chemotherapy with antimetabolites also causes such changes, with macrocytosis in the peripheral blood film.

2.1.2. Loss of red blood cells occurs as a result of bleeding, haemolysis or 'hypersplenism'. Bleeding (acute or chronic) is common in malignancy either from the tumour itself (particularly gastro-intestinal and bladder) or from an acquired haemorrhagic diathesis (see section 5).

Auto-immune haemolysis may be a feature of recurrence in some malignant conditions (particularly in lymphoid malignancy and to a lesser extent with carcinomas) and in widespread disease may rarely be due to microan-

Hancock, B. W. (ed.), Assessment of Tumour Response.
 ISBN 90-247-2712-X.
Printed in The Netherlands.

Table 1. Anaemia seen in the follow-up of cancer

Type	Indices	Investigations		
		Blood	Marrow	Others
Deficiency				
Iron deficient	Microcytic/Hypochromic	Iron↓ Iron binding capacity↑ Ferritin↓	Iron↓	Check diet and bleeding
Megaloblastic	Macrocytic/Normochromic	Folate↓(B12↓)	Megaloblastic	Exclude chemotherapy
Loss of red blood cells				
Bleeding – Acute	Normocytic/Normochromic	Retics↑	Erythroid hyperplasia	
Bleeding – Chronic	Microcytic/Hypochromic	Iron deficiency	Non-specific	Find source
Haemolysis – Immune	Normo (Macro) cytic/ Normochromic	Retics↑ Coombs +ve Haptoglobins↓ Bilirubin↑ Spherocytes ±	Erythroid hyperplasia	Steroid response
Haemolysis – Microangiopathic	Normocytic/Normochromic	Evidence of DIC Fragmented erythrocytes	Erythroid hyperplasia	Exclude sepsis
Hypersplenism	Normocytic/Normochromic	Pancytopenia	Erythroid hyperplasia	Spleen uptake scans +ve
Defective bone marrow				
Chronic disease	Normocytic/Normochromic	Iron↓ Iron binding capacity↓ Ferritin↑	Normal or hypoplastic	No response to iron therapy
Infiltration	Normocytic/Normochromic	Leucoerythroblastic film (later)	Malignant cells	Bone scan
Sideroblastic	Normochromic/Hypochromic	Iron↑ Iron binding capacity↓	Ring sideroblasts	
Myelosuppression (therapy induced)	Normocytic/Normochromic	Pancytopenia	Hypoplastic	

giopathic haemolytic anaemia in association with disseminated intravascular coagulation (see section 5).

In a large series of cases of auto-immune haemolytic anaemia (AIHA) presented from the Regional Blood Transfusion Centre, Sheffield [2] the antibody was usually of 'warm' type in chronic lymphocytic leukaemia, but with non-Hodgkin's lymphoma, Hodgkin's disease and carcinoma 'cold' antibodies were nearly as frequent and some cases showed features of 'warm' and 'cold' AIHA (so-called 'mixed' type). With the direct antiglobulin test positive reactions with antisera to IgG $\pm$ complement were usual in warm AIHA, to complement alone in cold AIHA and to IgG $\pm$ complement in mixed AIHA.

Hypersplensim may also develop in the course of malignant disease; a full discussion of this follows later (section 7).

2.1.3. Defective bone marrow production. The commonest type of anaemia seen during the follow-up of patients is that due to defective bone marrow production of red cells; often this is due to the non-specific 'toxic' effects of the chronic disease with associated block of reticulo-endothelial iron release. Infiltration by tumour cells and (of course) therapy induced myelosuppression are also major problems. In such patients the blood film may not be helpful; it is often simply normocytic/normochromic; bone marrow examination may give the answer but frequently the anaemia progresses (often requiring repeated transfusions) and the cause is not found until more overt evidence of recurrent disease is seen. Leucoërythroblastic anaemia describes the anaemia resulting from infiltration of the bone marrow by foreign or abnormal tissue; it is seen in metastatic malignant disease (particularly in tumours metastasising early to bone i.e. breast, bronchus, kidney, thyroid, prostate) and is characterised by the occurrence of immature white and red cells in the peripheral blood.

Sideroblastic anaemia is relatively uncommon but may be a cause of refractory anaemia at follow-up. A dimorphic (hypochromic/normochromic) picture is seen in the peripheral blood but marrow examination shows the presence of normoblasts containing an excess of iron granules particularly in ring distribution in the perinuclear mitochondria ('ring' sideroblasts). Such an anaemia may be a feature of any malignant condition but is particularly a feature of the myeloproliferative disorders.

2.2. Erythrocytosis/polycythaemia

Erythrocytosis (see ref. 2 for review) is the term used to describe the high red cell values found in certain diseases. Relative erythrocytosis is seen where red cell values (haemoglobin concentration, packed cell volume and red cell count) are mildly elevated in the absence of significantly increased red cell mass; it is seen in association with vascular disease particularly where the patient is a heavy smoker. Secondary erythrocytosis, where the red cell mass is elevated but in the absence of increased white cell and platelet counts (as in relative erythrocytosis) is not uncommonly seen during the follow-up of patients with cancer – it may be compensatory due to chronic lung or cardiac disease or may occur with inappropriate erythropoietin elaboration with disorders of kidney perfusion (cysts and hydronephrosis) and in association with some tumours where ectopic secretion of erythropoietic stimulating hormones similar to erythropoietin may occur (hypernephroma, hepatoma, cerebellar haemangioblastoma, uterine myofibroma, certain ovarian tumours). Tumour erythrocytosis is usually of mild degree and requires no specific treatment.

Erythrocytosis is also occasionally seen during follow-up of patients who have received androgenic steroids as part of their therapy.

Polycythaemia rubra vera, as distinct from erythrocytosis, is a myeloproliferative disorder involving benign proliferation of haemopoietic cells and is characterised by increased activity of white cell and platelet precursers as well as erythroid hyperplasia; red cell volume is increased and splenomegaly common. Thrombotic/haemorrhagic complications occur and treatment of the disorder is usually necessary.

3. White blood cell abnormalities

3.1. Leucocytosis

A problem occasionally encountered in the follow-up of the cancer patient is the so-called leukaemoid reaction. Extremely high (up to $50 \times 10^9/l$) white counts can be seen either as a manifestation of metastatic malignancy or less often as a response to infection, usually bacterial. The leukaemoid reaction differs from granulocytic leukaemia in that the cell count is usually below $50 \times 10^9/l$, that splenomegaly is absent, that other haemopoietic elements are often normal, that leucocyte alkaline phosphatase is usually high and that chromosomal studies are normal.

Eosinophilia, monocytosis and basophilia may also be seen in patients with neoplasm. All are particular features of Hodgkin's disease; eosinophilia and monocytosis may also be found in myeloproliferative disorders and in carcinoma whereas basophilia is not usually found in carcinoma. The mechanism of such abnormalities is unknown. Neutrophilia is also seen with steroid administration.

3.2.. Leucopenia

This is most often seen during follow-up as a result of cytotoxic chemotherapy or radiotherapy; it is now acknowledged that such myelosuppression may persist for months and even years (particularly after extensive or combined treatments). Lymphopenia per se is seen, in the absence of therapy effect, in patients with lymphomas (particularly Hodgkin's disease) and may carry a poor prognosis. Neutropenia in malignancy, if not due to therapy, may be due to decreased production ('toxic' or marrow infiltration) or from shortened survival (auto-immune or in association with hypersplenism).

4. Platelet abnormalities

4.1. Thrombocytosis

This is a common but unexplained feature of malignant disease [3]; it is found with solid tumours and with Hodgkin's disease and is often a marker of widespread disease. The platelet count in such patients may be used as a marker of disease response or recurrence but the megakaryocytic depression seen after therapy can complicate this assessment. Also it may be difficult to differentiate the high platelet count of malignancy from that seen with infection or acute bleeding; post-splenectomy thrombocytosis (in Hodgkin's disease) must also be kept in mind. The platelets of the thrombocytosis of malignancy usually have normal morphology and function (except in myeloproliferative and plasma cell dyscrasias) and it seems unlikely that this is a major cause of venous thrombosis in cancer. Thrombocytosis may also occur after the administration of certain drugs, particularly steroids and less often with vincristine.

4.2. Thrombocytopenia

When this is seen in the follow-up of patients with cancer it is most often a consequence of myelosuppressive therapy; if not, then the second most likely cause is infiltration of the bone marrow by tumour. Less frequently hypersplenism or autoimmune (immunologic) thrombocytopenia, usually in association with lymphoid malignancy, are found. Thrombocytopenia as a result of therapy is often associated with depression of the haemoglobin level and white cell count and the bone marrow is generally hypoplastic; the platelets function less actively than newly formed platelets and spontaneous bleeding can occur at counts below $20-30 \times 10^9/l$. In immunologic thrombocytopenia the platelet count alone is affected, the bone marrow shows active megakaryopoeisis, platelet antibodies may be demonstrated and since the peripheral platelets are young and functionally more active bleeding occurs only with counts much below $10 \times 10^9/l$.

4.3. Thrombocytopathy

Platelet function (aggregation, adhesion or the release reaction) may be impaired in certain malignant conditions, mainly macroglobulinaemia and other dysproteinaemias; it is believed that abnormal paraprotein coats the platelets thus depressing their function.

5. Immune function

A major problem in following patients with cancer is their susceptibility to infection; this results from the profound immunological disturbances which accompany the malignant condition (particularly when the lymphoreticular system is primarily involved or where there is widely disseminated tumour) and its therapy (with surgery, radiotherapy and cytotoxic drugs).

The immune response depends on complex interactions between lymphocytes, mononuclear phagocytes, antibody and complement and defects in any of these components may occur in cancer.

Neutrophil function which may be enhanced in untreated cancer patients [4] is, however, impaired in acute leukaemia and therapy (particularly chemotherapy) undoubtedly depresses the quality and quantity of neutrophil granulocytes; such patients are particularly prone to bacterial infection (including normal commensal organisms) but infection may not be well localised and pus formation is impaired. Most commonly these infections occur where host defence membrane barriers are broken (skin, gastro-intestinal, respiratory, genito-urinary).

Humoral immunity (B cell dependent) defects occur classically in myelomatosis, chronic lymphocytic leukaemia and after cytotoxic chemotherapy. Inadequate antibody production results in infection with organisms such as staphylococcus, streptococcus, pneumococcus, enterococci, and pneumocystis. Humoral immune defects may be potentiated by splenectomy in Hodgkin's disease [5].

One of the most important immune system interactions is between T cells and mononuclear phagocytic cells, disturbances in one causing abnormal function in the other. Macrophage function (see ref. 6 for review) may be enhanced (showing increased tumour cell cytotoxicity and bactericidal activity) in early malignancy but as the tumour disseminates, function is depressed, probably by circulating tumour cell products, e.g. sialoglycoproteins, prostaglandins, immune complexes. Successful treatment of the tumour would therefore be expected to restore immune function but this is complicated by the effects of the immunosuppressive agents, particularly chemotherapy, used in the treatment of the tumour [7].

The *in vitro* assessment of T cell function is notoriously difficult to interpret in the clinical situation; it does, however, appear that function is normal in localised malignancy but with widespread disease marked defects occur; this is particularly true of Hodgkin's disease [8].

The T cell immunosuppressive effects of therapy (particularly cytotoxic chemotherapy) are well recognised and this makes the follow-up assessment of immunity, in theory an excellent marker for assessing remission, non-response and relapse, difficult to interpret.

Patients with defects predominantly in the mononuclear phagocytic/T cell (cell mediated) part of the immune response tend to get infections with facultative or obligate intracellular parasites. Mycobacteria, cryptococcus, candida, pneumocystis, cytomegalovirus, varicella/zoster, and herpes simplex are the usual offenders.

Defects in immunity undoubtedly persist for up to a year after therapy though the incidence of infection decreases with time; in fact our recent studies [9] of patients with Hodgkin's disease reassessed 5 years following therapy show persistent depression of their lymphocyte transformation responses and of antibody levels.

6. Coagulation

It has long been recognised that there is an increased tendency to thrombotic conditions in neoplastic disease and this may occur independently of local involvement or compression by the tumour itself. Trousseau's syndrome, characteristically a recurrent migrating thrombophlebitis involving multiple sites, is particularly associated with cancer of the pancreas, lung, stomach and ovary. The cause of this thrombotic tendency has been variously ascribed to release of thromboplastic substances, alterations in coagulation factors, thrombocytosis, increased platelet adhesiveness, increased fibrinogen deposition, decreased fibrinolysis and increased fibrinogen deposition. It now seems likely that the most important mechanism is disseminated intravascular coagulation, DIC [10]. Patients with this syndrome in malignancy may have migrating thrombophlebitis, arterial embolisation (with or without thrombotic non-bacterial endocarditis) and haemorrhagic phenomena, depending upon the degree of coagulopathy. The syndrome is probably initiated by release of thromboplastic and proteolytic substances from cancer cells. Acute DIC in cancer, sometimes associated with severe sepsis, will result in serious clinical manifestations (purpura fulminans) and marked haematological abnormalities; low grade on-going DIC, usually associated with widespread or progressive cancer, results in large vessel thrombosis and the only obvious haematological abnormality may be that of elevated fibrinogen degradation products.

Hyperviscosity may also exacerbate a tendency to thrombosis or haemorrhage; this usually accompanies neoplasms with associated dysproteinaemia (particularly plasma cell dyscrasias) where the excess protein interferes with platelet function or myeloproliferative syndromes (such as polycythaemia vera) where platelet function is intrinsically abnormal.

7. Erythrocyte sedimentation rate (ESR)

The ESR is elevated when red cell rouleaux formation is enhanced. Rouleaux formation is controlled mainly by the concentrations of certain plasma proteins, particularly fibrinogen and to a lesser extent α_2 and γglobulins and glycoproteins. It is a completely non-specific test and a normal ESR does not exclude organic disease. In cancer the ESR is often elevated, particularly with widespread disease; in some neoplasms it can be a valuable prognostic marker when assessed prior to treatment. In malignant lymphoma, for example, an ESR of above 50 mm/h is usually associated with widespread disease and poor response to treatment [11]. Successful treatment of a neoplasm usually leads to a fall in the ESR; conversely a persistently elevated ESR or elevation after a period of normality is generally a marker of residual or recurrent tumour, having excluded, of course, intercurrent or coincidental disease, e.g. infection in that patient. The ESR may also become transiently elevated following intensive cytotoxic therapy (radiotherapy or chemotherapy) presumably due to reactive changes in plasma proteins occurring as a result of the breakdown of tumour and normal tissue cells. Anaemia itself may also cause elevation of the ESR by altering the ratio of red cells to plasma, thus encouraging rouleaux formation; since anaemia is common in malignancy it should be excluded before attributing the high ESR solely to neoplasm. The ESR also increases with age and values of above 20 mm/h in the absence of organic disease are seen in older patients.

Plasma viscosity generally parallels the ESR but is less affected by anaemia and age; it is dependent on the plasma concentration of macromolecular proteins. It is however less convenient and more expensive to measure than the ESR.

8. The spleen

Since the spleen is the largest lymphoid organ in the body it commonly obtrudes on the management of patients with malignant disease. The particular problems are: a) whether or not it is palpable; b) whether splenic enlargement is due to infiltration by disease; c) the spleen as a cause of pain; d) hypersplenism; e) when the spleen should be removed; f) the consequences of splenectomy; and g) the entity, hyposplenism.

8.1. Splenic enlargement

If the spleen can be easily palpated, it is probably at least three times normal size unless it is being displaced by a space-occupying lesion, e.g. a suprarenal tumour. When there is doubt it is valuable to have the position clarified by a soft tissue radiograph or a spleen scan.

In the context of malignant disease, very large spleens are only seen in chronic granulocytic leukaemia, myeloid metaplasia and some types of non-Hodgkin's lymphoma. Moderate enlargement of the spleen can be encountered in all varieties of leukaemia and lymphoma. Primary tumours of the spleen are excessively rare; the only important one is the haemangioma of which about one-third of the few reported cases have been malignant. Metastatic spread of carcinoma to the spleen is also uncommon but it has been described in carcinoma of breast and bronchus and in malignant melanoma.

Not all palpable spleens in patients with malignant disease are infiltrated with neoplastic cells. Apart from being displaced by extrasplenic tumours, they may be enlarged for a variety of reasons. It has been shown from staging laparotomies in Hodgkin's disease that about 25% of palpable spleens merely show lymphoreticular hyperplasia consistent with an immunological reaction to the tumour; although not documented this could occur in other forms of cancer. Congestive splenomegaly may arise from portal or splenic vein thrombosis due to contiguous disease, e.g. pancreas. Myeloid metaplasia (extra-medullary haemopoiesis) can occur in disseminated carcinomatosis with widespread bone marrow involvement.

The spleen has a rich arterial blood supply and high blood flow. However, the branching arterioles within the spleen do not anastomose and peripheral infarction with perisplenitis is seen commonly in splenomegaly from all causes.

8.2. Hypersplenism

The term hypersplenism (see ref. 12 for review) has caused confusion. It is best confined to depression of peripheral blood counts due to splenic enlargement. The effect may be seen on any or all of the blood elements and if for any reason the spleen is removed the blood counts will improve. Hypersplenism can be seen in the presence of a normal or hyperplastic bone marrow or it may compound depressed marrow function due to infiltration by disease or the effects of therapy. It has long been postulated that hypersplenism is due to a humoral factor secreted by the spleen which has a 'braking' effect on the marrow, an effect enhanced by splenic enlargement. There are some clinical and experimental observations which support such a thesis but the fact is that no humoral factor has ever been isolated from the splenic substance or the splenic venous outflow. The entity hypersplenism can be satisfactorily explained by a combination of factors that have now been demonstrated in splenomegaly from different causes. First, there is a variable degree of 'pooling' of cells outwith the circulation in the lymphatic cords of the spleen; the extent of this correlates well with spleen size. Second, there is an element of blood cell dilution due to expansion of the plasma volume analogous to that seen in pregnancy; again this correlates well with spleen size. The reason for this hypervolaemia is obscure; probably the blood volume has to increase to fill the vascular space in the splanchnic bed and enlarged spleen; the marrow's ability to expand the red cell volume is limited and the plasma volume therefore increases disproportionately. Third, it has been shown for red cells at least that there may be reduction of the cell survival time. When there is a marrow defect as well as splenic enlargement it can be very difficult to assess the relative contribution of splenomegaly to cytopenia.

8.3. Splenectomy

The reasons for splenectomy in patients with malignant disease are few. Obviously the spleen should be removed if it is suspected that the patient has a primary splenic tumour. It is justified if marked hypersplenism is suspected and the spleen size cannot be reduced by specific cancer therapy; it sometimes arises that severe neutropenia is in the background of recurrent infections or thrombocytopenia is causing troublesome bleeding or the patient is requiring very frequent blood transfusions. Splenectomy is considered in the presence of autoimmune haemolytic anaemia or immune thrombocytopenia that is not responding to corticosteroids and specific antitumour therapy.

Occasionally splenectomy is undertaken when the spleen is very large and causing mechanical disconfort or is the site of frequent infarction. By far the most frequent reason for removing the spleen at the present time is as part of the staging process in the initial assessment of some patients with Hodgkin's disease.

Although the spleen can be removed with relative impunity in a majority of individuals, splenectomy cannot be dismissed as a benign procedure. The effects are several. Immediately after operation there is a leucocytosis and thrombocytosis. The platelet count can rise to more than 1000×10^9/l and there is a temporary danger of thrombosis; it is wise to insist on early ambulation and to use platelet anti-aggregating drugs (e.g. aspirin and dipyridamole) until the platelet count falls to below 500×10^9/l. Although these elevated counts usually settle after 2–3 weeks they may stay up indefinitely. For the rest of the patient's life the peripheral blood will show malformed red cells and red cells with inclusions, e.g. Howell-Jolly bodies and iron granules (siderocytes). The most important concern is the proneness to infection. This is probably explained because the spleen is a significant filter and organ of phagocytosis and is concerned with the secondary immune response. Levels of IgM tend to fall after splenectomy and may not rise appropriately to an infective challenge particularly if the patient has received intensive chemotherapy. The infective risk is unpredictable but it is worst in very young children, in patients who are immunodepressed because of extensive disease and in patients immunodepressed because of their treatment.

One incidental result of splenectomy is that when there is a cause for reticulocytosis or leucocytosis the response is abnormally high.

3.4. Hyposplenism

Hyposplenism (see ref. 13 for review) is a relatively new term which is not the opposite of hypersplenism. It has come to be used when the blood shows mis-shapen red cells and red cells with inclusions (as after splenectomy) due to splenic atrophy. The splenic shrinkage can be confirmed using spleen scanning techniques and functional deficiency can be demonstrated by the delayed clearance of heat damaged radioactive labelled red cells. There is evidence that patients showing the blood changes of hyposplenism may also have a degree of immunodeficiency and proneness to infection.

In the context of malignant disease, hyposplenism might be encountered in rare circumstances. It is seen in intestinal malabsorption (adult coeliac disease) and ulcerative colitis and therefore might be seen when these gut disorders are complicated by neoplasia. It is also seen when the spleen infarcts due to arterial thrombosis in essential thrombocythaemia.

9. Iron, ferritin, folate and vitamin B12

9.1. Iron

A number of measurements of iron metabolism are disturbed by malignant disease. A low serum iron level with expansion of the total iron binding capacity (TIBC) is significant of iron deficiency. Otherwise changes in the serum iron and TIBC are too non-specific to be of diagnostic value. The TIBC is commonly depressed when malignant disease is in relapse. The serum iron may be low with extensive disease. Raised serum iron levels occur in marrow hypoplasia, after multiple transfusions (in the absence of bleeding), in sideroblastic anaemia and in patients with extensive liver involvement.

9.2. Ferritin

The serum ferritin on the other hand may prove to have value in the assessment of disease status. Ferritin is a ubiquitous protein found in all types of cells (see ref. 14 for review). Its principal function is to act as a store or reserve of iron, which can be utilised for haem synthesis, and it may donate its iron directly to mitochondria for this purpose. Its storage function also provides a means by which cellular iron levels are kept low, thereby circumventing the potential toxicity of iron. The storage mechanism includes the stimulation by iron of the biosynthesis of ferritin protein (apoferritin), which then acts as a cage to entrap further iron entering the cell. Ferritin is predominantly located intracellularly but the development of sensitive radioimmunoassays has established that minute quantities are normally present in the serum, (see ref. 15 for review). In normal, healthy individuals the concentration of serum ferritin is usually directly related to the size of iron stores; in patients with iron deficiency and iron overload, alterations in reticuloendothelial (RE) iron content are followed by changes in serum ferritin concentration. Repeated venesection results in a decrease in iron stores and fall in serum ferritin; with administration of iron orally or parenterally the serum ferritin level rises.

Serum ferritin distinguishes between absolute iron deficiencies, as seen with blood or dietary deficiency (low serum ferritin) and the disturbance of the RE system with blocked release of iron, as occurs in 'chronic' disease (normal or increased serum ferritin). Such information from a simple test may be helpful in establishing the cause of an anaemia occurring during the follow-up of a patient with malignancy. However, elevated serum ferritin, apart from that seen with non-specific anaemia, RE iron malutilization, and tissue damage, may also result from tumour production of the protein. In leukaemic patients, elevated serum ferritin is derived from circulating leucocytes [16], and elevated levels in patients with germ cell tumours correlate well with response to therapy and may be useful in the early detection of recurrent or residual tumour disease [17]. In malignant lymphoma a percentage of patients are sensitized to ferritin purified from spleens involved by Hodgkin's disease, but not to normal splenic ferritin [18]. The existence of tumour-specific ferritin is further supported by changes from the normal isoferritin phenotype in neoplastic tissue. It has been suggested that there are specific 'carcinofoetal' isoferritins, immunologically similar to heart ferritins, and that serum ferritin might therefore sometimes have a role as a tumour marker [19].

9.3. Folate

Since folate has a biological half-life of only a few weeks in the body and is readily destroyed by cooking, disturbance of folate metabolism manifests itself relatively quickly. The first indications are macrocytosis and hypersegmentation of the peripheral blood neutrophils and then of course megaloblastic change in the bone marrow.

There are several possible reasons for interference with folate nutrition in cancer. Folate deficiency may be seen in a few weeks if there is marked loss of appetite or dysphagia. Extensive infiltrative disease of the small intestine affects folic acid absorption. Any rapidly dividing tumour, particularly if complicated by haemolysis and particularly in a malnourished person, may quickly give rise to conditioned folate depletion. The unique problem affecting folic acid in malignant disease is the frequent use of the antimetabolite, methotrexate, as a therapeutic agent. Methotrexate inhibits cell division because it antagonises dihydrofolate reductase; in some treatment schedules the dose of methotrexate is such that megaloblastic anaemia is inevitable unless the use of methotrexate is followed by 'folinic acid rescue'.

9.4. Vitamin B12

Because the daily requirement for vitamin B12 is very low and the biological half-life very long (about one year) nutritional deficiency of vitamin B12 is unlikely to occur as a direct result of malignant disease. Malabsorption will occur due to intrinsic factor deficiency after total gastrectomy for neoplastic disease and megaloblastic anaemia may develop early due to previous atrophic gastritis. Malabsorption of vitamin B12 also occurs if there is extensive disease of the terminal ileum or if there is resection or bypass of the ileum.

It is not widely known that anomalous results for serum vitamin B12 values may be obtained in some of the myeloproliferative syndromes. There are two main vitamin B12 transport proteins in the plasma, transcobalamin I and transcobalamin II; binding protein has also been found in erythrocytes, lymphocytes and in high concentrations in mature granulocytes. It has been reported that in chronic granulocytic leukaemia and in myeloid metaplasia with raised leucocyte counts, the serum vitamin B12 level may be greatly elevated; this is due particularly to elevation of transcobalamin I. A third binding protein related to the transcobalamin I complex has been identified and termed transcobalamin III; its function is uncertain but elevated levels have been found in patients with polycythaemia rubra vera.

References

1. Sokol RJ, Hewitt S, Stamps BK: Autoimmune haemolysis: an 18 year study of 865 cases referred to a Regional Transfusion Centre. Br Med J 282:2023–2027, 1981.
2. Penington D: Erythrocytosis and myeloproliferative disorders. Medicine (UK) 29:1513–1517, 1980.
3. Levin J, Conley CL: Thrombocytosis associated with malignant disease. Arch Intern Med 114:497–500, 1964.
4. Bruce L, Hancock BW, Richmond J: Neutrophil function in human malignant disease. J Physiol 259:48–50 p, 1976.
5. Hancock BW, Bruce L, Dunsmore IR, Milford Ward A, Richmond J: Follow-up studies on the immune status of patients with Hodgkin's disease after splenectomy and treatment, in relapse and remission. Br J Cancer 36:347–354, 1977.
6. Dent RG: The role of the mononuclear phagocyte system in cancer. Hosp Update 6, 469–479, 1980.
7. McVie JG: Secondary immunosuppression. In: 'Cancer assessment and monitoring', Symmington T, Williams AE, McVie JG (eds). Edinburgh: Churchill Livingstone, 1980, pp 120–136.
8. Hancock BW, Bruce L, Sugden P, Milford Ward A, Richmond J: Immune status in patients with untreated malignant lymphoma – a multifactorial study. Clin Oncol 3:57–63, 1977.
9. Hancock BW, Bruce L, Whitham MD, Ward AM, Richmond J: Immunity in Hodgkin's disease, five years after treatment – a follow-up study. In press Br J Cancer.
10. Sack GH, Levin J, Bell WR: Trousseau's syndrome and other manifestations of chronic disseminated coagulapathy in patients with neoplasms: clinical, pathophysiologic and therapeutic features. Medicine 56:1–37, 1977.
11. Hancock BW, May K, Bruce L, Dunsmore IR, Clarke A, Milford Ward A: Haematological and immunological markers in malignant lymphoma. Tumor Diagnostik 1:140–144, 1980.
12. Richmond J: Hypersplenism. Br J Hosp Med 24:405–412, 1980.
13. Bullen AW, Losowsky MS: Consequences of impaired splenic function. Clin Sci 57:129–137, 1979.
14. Harrison PM: Ferritin, an iron storage molecule. Semin Haematol 14:55–70, 1977.
15. Jacobs A, Worwood M: Ferritin in serum. N Engl J Med 292:951–956, 1975.
16. White GP, Worwood M, Parry DH, Jacobs A: Ferritin synthesis in normal and leukaemic leucocytes. Nature 250:584–586, 1974.
17. Grail A, Bates J, Milford Ward A, Hancock BW: Serum ferritin as a third marker in germ cell tumours. Eur J Cancer 18:261–269, 1982.
18. Hancock BW, Bruce L, May K, Richmond J: Ferritin, a sensitising substance in the leucocyte migration inhibition test in patients with malignant lymphoma. Br J Haematol 43:223–233, 1979.
19. Hazard JT, Drysdale JW: Ferritinaemia in cancer. Nature 265:755–756, 1977.

7. Pathological Assessment

C. M. D. ROSS

1. Introduction

The role of the tissue pathologist in the management of neoplastic disease is principally that of determining that a neoplastic process is present, of establishing the nature of the disease and of assessing those characteristics that may be of predictive value. Since the sensitivity of various neoplasms to different forms of therapy is broadly established, these pathological observations can be helpful in guiding management.

When surgery is used other pathological observations are required to determine the probability of clearance of the growth, to identify vascular permeation with the implications for metastasis and to detect nodal metastases.

The same criteria are important when assessing material submitted during or after treatment of the primary lesion(s) but the histological features may be influenced at this stage by both the effects of treatment and by changes in the behaviour of the tumour itself with the passage of time.

2. Histological assessment of tumour response

Over the past 40 years or so, several attempts have been made to identify tumour responses to radiation that would be helpful in assessing probable outcome [1–9].

Ideally, sampling of tumours with the intention of examining the effects of treatment should not appreciably disturb patients. Consequently most studies have been concerned with carcinoma of the cervix where the growth is readily accessible and where the occasions of insertion of radioactive applications afford a convenient opportunity for repeated biopsy. The growing edge of the tumour is sampled to try to avoid already dead and unresponsive tissue. If sequential biopsies are taken, a clock-face notation can be used so that neighbouring foci are examined. Apart from the pre-irradiation diagnostic biopsy, specimens are usually taken about a week after the start of irradiation with possible further sampling 1–3 weeks later (see Figs. 1a, b, 2a, b).

Hancock, B. W. (ed.), Assessment of Tumour Response.

ISBN 90-247-2712-X.
Printed in The Netherlands.

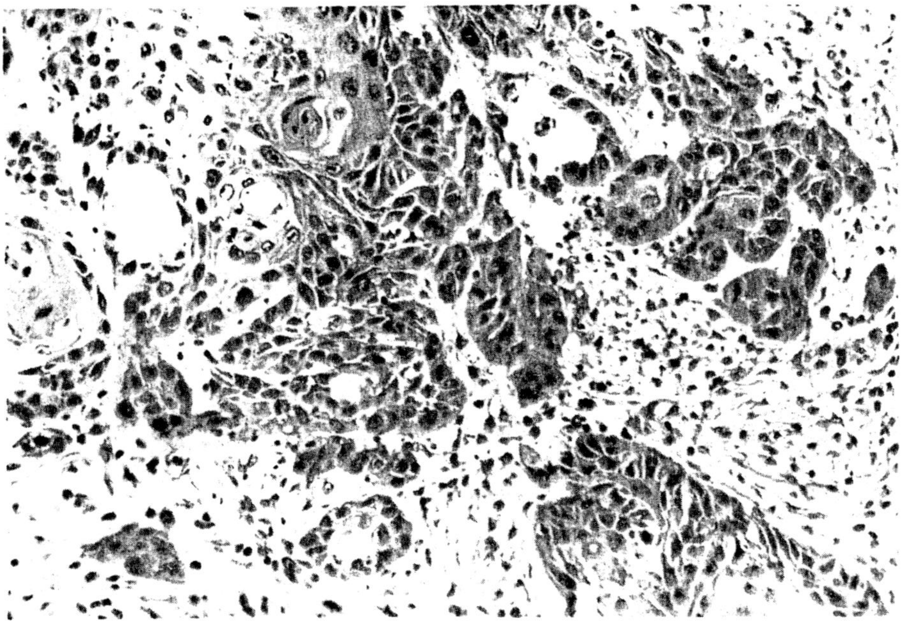

Figure 1a. Squamous cell carcinoma, cervix uteri (haematoxylin and eosin, H & E).

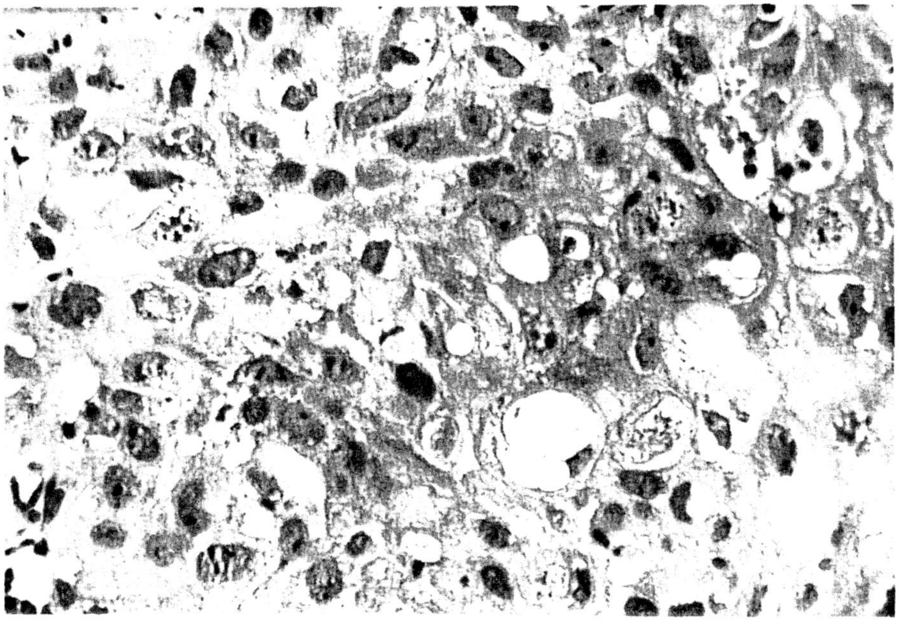

Figure 1b. Same tumour after first application of radio-active caesium, showing marked degenerative change (H & E).

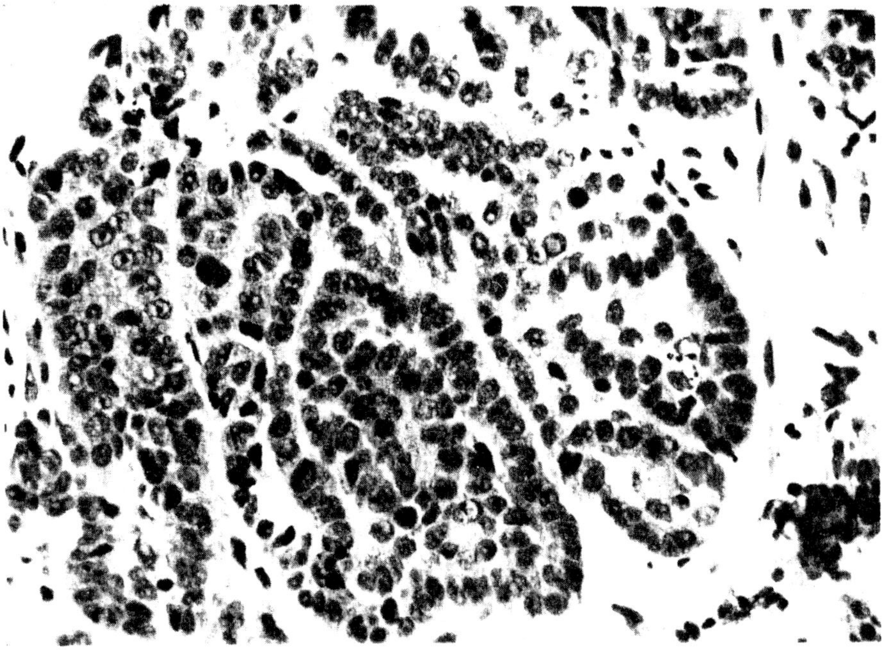

Figure 2a. Adenocarcinoma of cervix uteri (H & E).

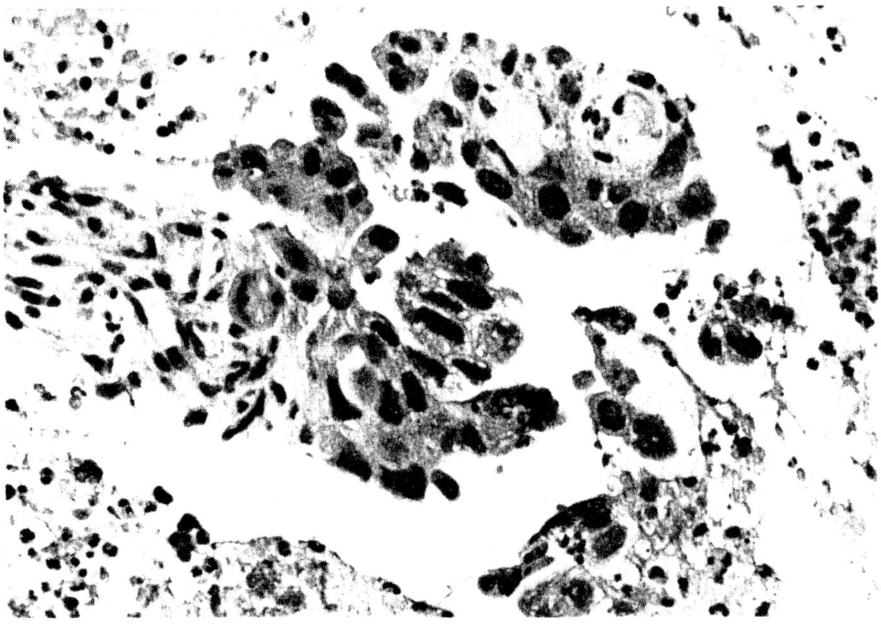

Figure 2b. Same tumour after first application of radio-active caesium. Degeneration, necrosis and inflammatory exudate are present (H & E).

The criteria considered to indicate a favourable response to radiation include:

1. Reduction in number of normal mitoses with an increase in abnormal, ineffective, mitoses.
2. Increase in cell size and increase in number of keratinising cells (differentiation). Mucous cells may become more numerous in adenocarcinoma.
3. Reduction in non-dividing, non differentiating, 'resting' or viable cells below 30% of the cell population at 7 days.
4. Increase in number of degenerate cells.

Glucksman and Way [4] classified dividing cells and resting cells (potential dividing cells) in group A and combined differentiating (mainly keratotic or parakeratotic) cells with degenerating cells in group B. Elimination of group A in favour of group B was thought favourable, with no normal mitoses and less that 3% resting cells 7 days after the commencement of treatment.

Gusberg [6] proposed categories A and B with essentially the same constituents but based assessment on DNA staining of nuclei which displayed a heavy chromatin pattern in viable cells of category A and relative dilution of DNA and prominence of nucleoli in category B.

Other findings such as the inflammatory response, necrosis and the presence of bizarre or multinuclear cells are not thought relevant.

These observations only relate to the local tumour. It is claimed [8, 9] that 5-year survival is significantly more likely in patients in stages I–III who show a good histological response.

Although not routinely assessed, capillary damage would be expected to influence outcome. It has been calculated that the critical distance between tumour cells and their blood supply is about 145 μ [10]. Vascular damage could cause necrosis of many cells within that range and may be responsible for the tumour bed effect experimentally displayed by depression of volume growth rate of tumours transplanted to previously irradiated sites in mice [11, 12].

Trott [13] suggests that the changes seen in favourable responders may relate to re-oxygenation and that the small proportion of neoplastic cells (1% or less) that are not promptly sterilised by irradiation may be rendered more susceptible by the use of high pressure oxygen in conjunction with radiotherapy, fast neutrons and hypoxic radiosensitisers in the case of apparently poor responders. He also remains convinced of the prognostic value of histological assessment.

A recent study of 116 cases of carcinoma of cervix included histological assessment using novel, but seemingly simple criteria [14]:

(1) No tumour seen;

(2) Tumour considered non-viable;

(3) Tumour doubtfully viable;
(4) Tumour viable.

It was concluded that histological assessment correlated poorly with outcome. Bearing in mind Trott's observation that 99% of tumour cells are killed in any case, this probably reflects irrelevance of the criteria.

Histology occasionally has a role in assessment of unusual therapeutic modalities. Intralesional inoculation as in the use of extracts of BCG or PPD has been shown to cause tumour disappearance in association with inflammatory cell infiltrate, necrosis or granulomata [15].

3. Late effects of treatment

Late sequelae of radiation include stromal changes with fibrosis, hyalinisation of collagen, focal necrosis and vessel wall thickening which may be associated with thrombosis. Hypoxia from this cause with reduction of fine vasculature may promote insensitivity to irradiation in any surviving neoplastic cells. Alternatively, necrosis of such cells may ensue. There may be many bizarre fibroblasts, often with large irregular nuclei and quite numerous mitoses, in granulation or scarring tissue. Such cells may have to be differentiated from residual malignant cells (Fig. 3).

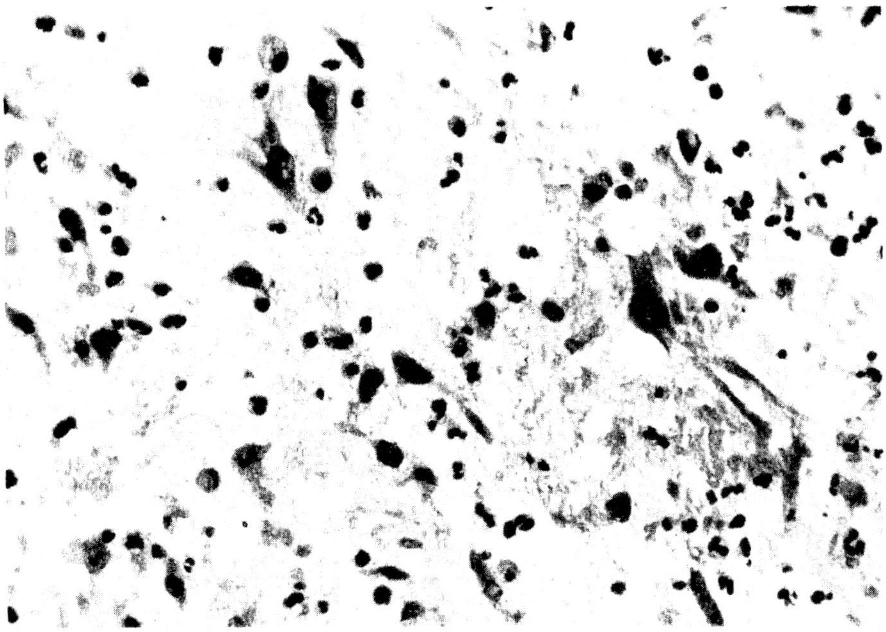

Figure 3. Granulation tissue from tracheostomy wound of patient treated by irradiation for carcinoma of larynx. Note bizarre giant nuclei of fibroblasts which have to be distinguished from neoplastic spread (H & E).

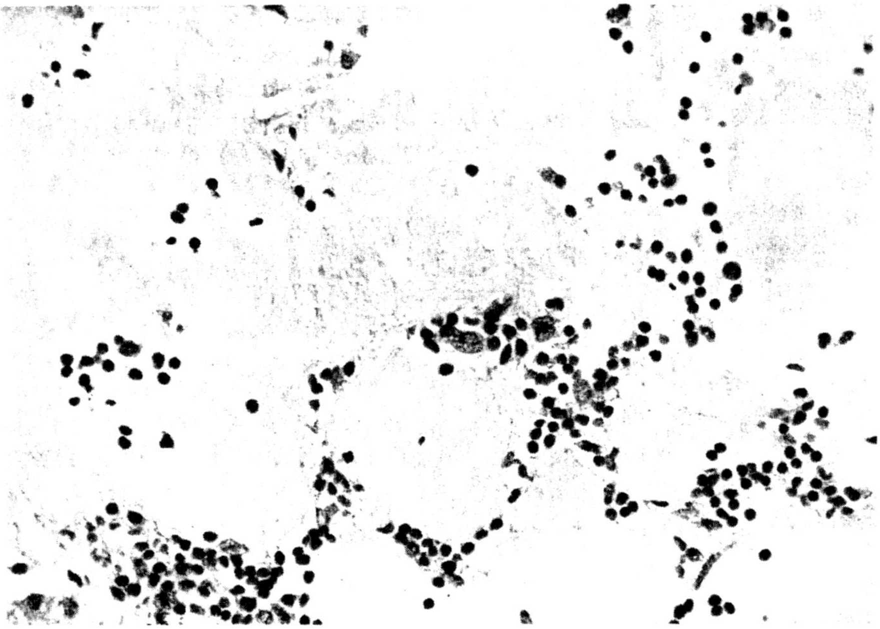

Figure 4. Hodgkin's disease following chemotherapy. There is much fibrosis, few lymphoid cells and no identifiable neoplastic cells (H & E).

Treatment of lymphomas produces depletion of lymphoid cells with eventual dense fibrosis so that all recognisable evidence of lymphoma may be lost (Fig. 4).

There are other aspects in which histological examination is useful in the later management of neoplastic disease. Where recurrence is indicated clinically by such features as nodular, ulcerated or granulomatous foci in the treated region, repeat biopsy is desirable. Metastases may be confirmed similarly.

Cellular atypia due to radiation may lead to erroneous diagnosis of extension of malignant disease. Altered mesothelial cells may be mistaken for Sternberg-Reed cells [16].

Apart from persisting or recurring, neoplasms may respond to irradiation by undergoing a change in character. For example, verrucous carcinoma rarely metastasises but, following irradiation, may become more aggressive and, on histological examination, show loss of differentiation [17–19].

4. Changes not attributable to treatment

It is common for neoplastic tissue to undergo such processes as necrosis, haemorrhage, ulceration or infection. Hodgkin's disease in its mixed cellularity form typically shows progressive necroses and fibrosis which may modify histological appearances, even without treatment. Fibrosis may greatly modify the appearance of the nodular sclerosis form of the disease.

Apart from events of this type, neoplasms may exhibit other forms of change which may, mistakenly, be thought to arise from therapy.

4.1. Tumour progression

This term relates to the development of new properties and may be manifested in various ways such as loss of hormonal dependence in breast or endocrine tumours, cytogenetic changes, enzyme pattern changes or increasing aggressiveness [20].

From the tissue pathologist's viewpoint histological changes may be found. It is common for metastases to be less differentiated than their parent tumour, although it is unlikely that such variation would be mistaken for therapeutic effect. Lymphomas tend to alter to more aggressive forms with the passage of time [21] and this may occur in patients under treatment.

The converse of progression is maturation in which growth assumes a less aggressive form with the passage of time. The best known example is the transformation of neuroblastoma to ganglioneuroblastoma and ganglioneuroma.

4.2. Spontaneous regression

Very occasionally, tumours regress and may even disappear in the absence of treatment [22].

The majority of examples comprise only four tumour types – renal cell carcinoma, neuroblastoma, melanoma and choriocarcinoma but breast, bladder, gonads and lymphoid tissue are established sources of other instances. In most cases, the phenomenon is confirmed clinically, usually with radiological evidence. Serological assay of tumour markers is of use where tumour type is appropriate, as in germ cell tumours.

However, confirmation of the phenomenon is dependent on biopsy of the growth with histological confirmation of its nature. The need for such tissue confirmation is even more important to establish the occurrence of abscopal regression, which is the regression of an untreated metastatic tumour following treatment of a primary growth. Such confirmation is seldom obtained [23–25] and even use of cytological examinations of effusions is not entirely convincing as an alternative [26].

5. Autopsy

Although autopsy examination is usually undertaken in selected cases, it is clearly worth consideration in that it allows unlimited access to determine the extent and location of disease.

Failure to find evidence of residual tumour is not uncommon and death may be found to be due to some other cause, possibly related to therapy, possibly entirely unconnected. Alternatively, relative or total treatment failure is assessable. Findings may be relevant to management of subsequent cases.

6. Cytological assessment of tumour response

Although cytological examination has diagnostic use in neoplasms of many sites, the cervix uteri is most commonly the target for this procedure. For this reason, attempts to assess radiosusceptibility before, or after the start of, irradiation have been based on cervical smears. In a series of papers [27–31], the Grahams described numerous features to be noted and offered two conceptually different proposals, the Sensitisation Response (SR) and the Radiation Response (RR).

The Sensitisation Response is based on features noted in a differential count of at least 100 non-neoplastic cells in smears from carcinoma of cervix. A favourable SR is indicated where (para)basal cells account for more than 10% of cells and where they show fine vacuolation, perhaps with red-staining granules, and increased cytoplasmic density. These characteristics are subtle and others have found it difficult to emulate the results of the Grahams. A high SR really implies a post-menopausal state.

Radiation Response is based on examination of smears a few days after the start of irradiation and, like SR, involves recognition of changes in non-malignant cells. Four features are sought:

1. Cytoplasmic vacuolation;
2. Cell enlargement by at least a third with concomitant nuclear enlargement;
3. Nuclear wrinkling and disarrangement of nuclear pattern;
4. Increased number of nuclei in individual cells.

Originally, the presence of bizarre cells was a fifth criterion, but paucity of such cells made this less useful.

It was claimed that RR exceeding 75% indicated a good prospect of radiocurability of the local tumour. Conversely, RR less than 60% implied a poor response.

Experience of others has been mixed. Recently, Agnew *et al.* [32] found quite good correlation but Rubio *et al.* [33] found both RR and SR of no value in a much larger series of cases. They cite 39 other papers which overall show a slight preponderance in which accord between RR and clinical outcome was poor.

A 'Cornification Index' has been suggested as a prognostic pointer [34]. The percentage of cornified cells among superficial and intermediate cells is about 5% in normal post-menopausal smears but usually more than 10% where cervical carcinoma is present. The use of this estimation for follow-up of treated cases was proposed.

It can be difficult to distinguish irradiated non-malignant cells from malignant cells and further difficulty in assessement may follow changes in cell distribution following irradiation. A method involving assessment of RR on irradiated normal buccal cells has, therefore, been suggested but not perpetuated [35].

As with histology, exfoliative cytology is useful in the recognition of recurrence or spread following definite therapy. Apart from smears taken from suspect surfaces, such as vagina, body fluids are often examined, either to recognise involvement by disseminated malignant cells or to evaluate response to treatment (Figs. 5, 6, 7).

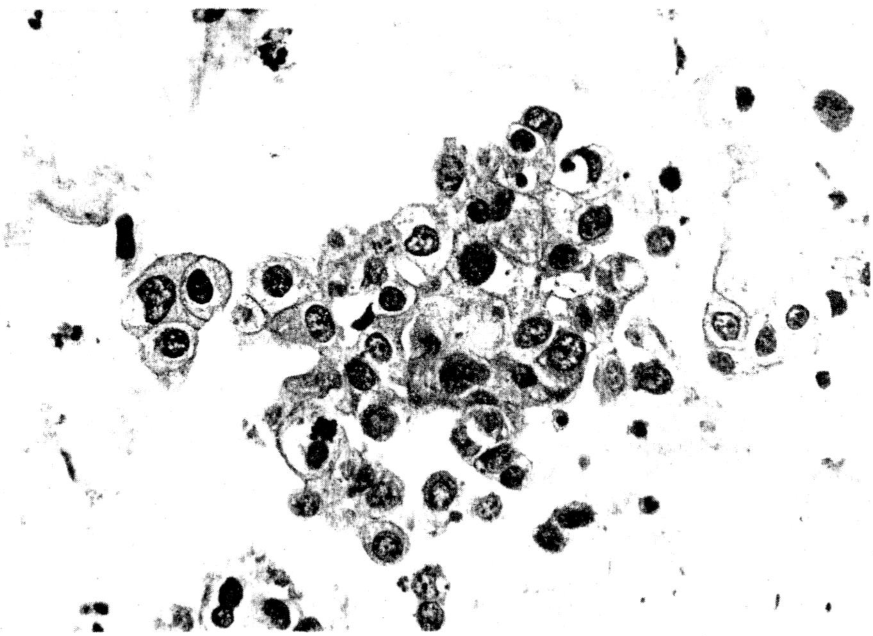

Figure 5. Urine – fragments of urothelial carcinoma (Papanicolaou).

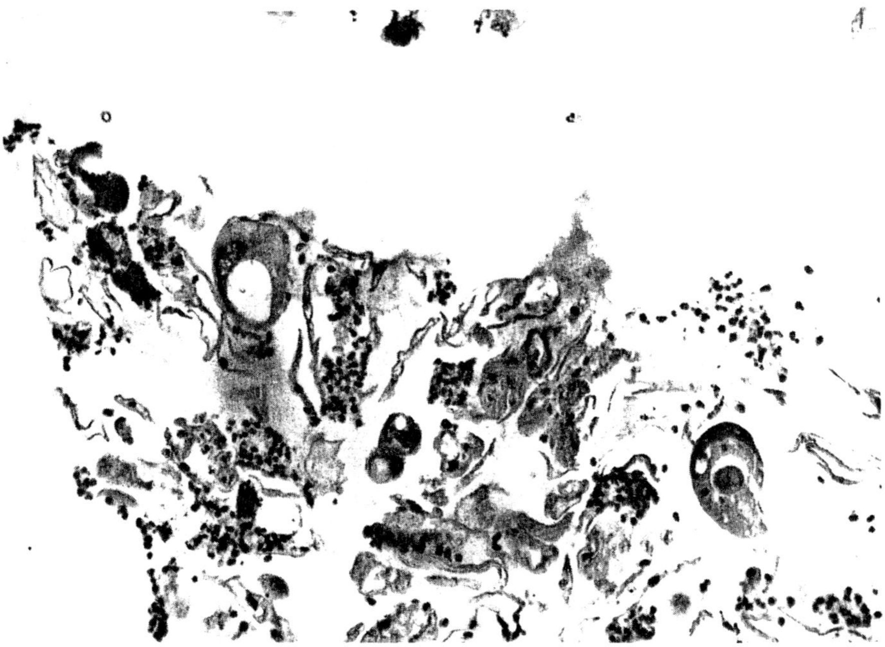

Figure 6. Same case following radiotherapy to bladder. There are enlarged bizarre vacuolated cells and loss of recognisable neoplastic cells (Papanicolaou).

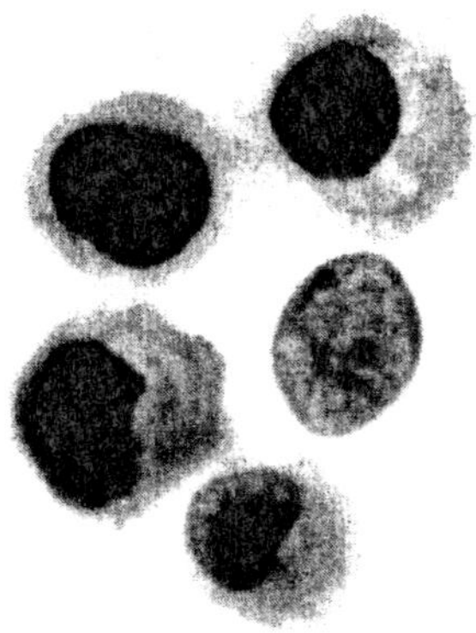

Figure 7. Cerebro-spinal fluid – metastatic breast carcinoma cells. These cells disappeared from the CSF following treatment.

7. Tumour chemistry

Estimation of DNA content using Feulgen staining or other techniques can be of value in determining the effect of therapy on a neoplasms and is considered under 'flow cytometry' (section 11).

Changes in tumour enzymes can be shown following treatment. For example, glycolysis enzymes measured in tissue homogenates of samples of cervical cancer have been shown to decrease but there was no correlation with clinical outcome or histological grade [36]. In an experimental rat tumour, a rise in nuclease, demonstrated by a lead nitrate technique, follows cyclophosphamide treatment [37] and it is suggested that this could be a useful technique in assessment of response.

8. Electron microscopy

So far, this has found little use in the study of clinical responses to treatment. The most striking specific effect that is demonstrable follows use of antitubulins such as vinca alkaloids. Damaged cells cannot form a spindle during cell division and lose their subplasmalemmal arrays of microtulules [38].

9. Experimental and new procedures

Histological and cytomorphological techniques have proved of limited or doubtful value and there is a dearth of recent studies based on such methods. It is useful, therefore, to consider those experimental methods which have been used to study mainly animal tumours and to note their applications to human tumours.

9.1. In vivo assays [39]

In general, these entail the use of xenografts in which neoplastic tissue is inoculated by various routes into experimental animals.

9.1.1. End-point dilution assay [40]. A suspension of single cells has to be prepared from the tumour under study and a range of dilutions injected subcutaneously or intramuscularly, usually into several sites in the host animals. The aim is to determine the number of tumour cells required to produce tumours at 50% of the inoculated sites (TD50).

This method allows assessment of the effects of different treatment modalities [41]. However, preparation of single cell suspensions from solid tumours is difficult, the test takes a long time and it uses many animals.

9.1.2. Tumour (growth) latency assay [42]. This obviates the necessity for single cell suspensions since it depends on determination of the delay in appearance of tumours in inoculated animals (latency period).

The response of treated tumours can be compared with untreated tumours to indicate the surviving fraction. Results can be influenced by a variety of associated factors [43].

9.1.3. Lung colony assay [44]. Like the end-point dilution assay, this requires preparation of single cell suspensions. Intravenous injection into recipient mice gives rise to microscopic nodules in the lungs within 16 to 20 days. Cloning efficiency can be calculated from a colony count. The ratio of cloning efficiency of treated and control tumours indicates the cell survival in treated tumours. This technique has the advantage of requiring fewer test animals and is also more rapid than the other procedure.

In vivo procedures are hedged with many variables. Apart from the need for controls, animals of low immunogenicity are required. Heavily irradiated cells added to the inoculum greatly increase the efficacy of transplantation [41, 45] and must be added to untreated controls since irradiated test tumours will contain numerous lethally irradiated cells.

These procedures are available for the study of human neoplasms using mice which are rendered immunologically deficient following thymectomy, usually followed by cytosine arabinoside and whole body irradiation [46–48]. Many types of tumours have been successfully transplanted including carcinomas of pancreas, large bowel, uterus and ovary as well as melanomas. Breast carcinomas are more difficult to establish [49].

Alternatively, and more expensively, nude mice [50, 51] or nude rats [52] can be used.

Because of the variations in 'take' of human tumours, these methods would be of limited value in assessing clonogenicity of individual cases. However, they can readily be applied to assessment of therapeutic response to various regimens.

9.2. In vitro assays

Tumour cells can be cultured in suitable media to determine clonogenicity in relation to therapy, analogously to *in vivo* end point dilution assay. This can be quicker and obviates the use of host animals as well.

However, human tumour cells usually exhibit low plating efficiency. A soft agar medium with a replaceable liquid component has been used to grow human pancreatic tumours but these were initially xenografted into suitable prepared mice [53, 54]. Such xenografts can be used for cytotoxic assay.

Human ovarian cancer cells from effusions have been grown directly in soft agar and sensitivity tested to doxorubicin, cis-platinum, melphalan and 5-fluorouracil [55, 56]. The factors that may modify the results of *in vitro* assay have recently been reviewed [57].

A variation involves growth of tumour cells in semi-solid agar to produce 'spheroids' which are morphologically likened to nodules of solid carcinomas and which have a heterogeneous cell population with hypoxic cells more deeply located [58]. Such spheroids provide a useful target for evaluation of cytotoxic agents [59].

10. Autoradiography

Methods used under this heading can be applied to assessment of cell kinetics in neoplasms. In principle, a radio-active base, usually tritiated thymidine or tritiated uridine, is injected intravascularly and several samples of the tumour under investigation are taken, either as incisional or punch biopsies or, more commonly, as aspirates. Smears or sections are stained by Feulgen's method to show DNA which is assessed by microdensitometry and are used to prepare autoradiographs [60–63].

The percentage of cell nuclei showing grains is counted to give a 'Labelling Index' and this gives a measure of the number of cells in S-phase at the time of administration of tritiated thymidine.

'Percent Labelled Mitoses' is determined from a count of 50–200 dividing cells. Cell cycle distributions can be estimated and, by using serial samples, a curve can be constructed to show the passage of the wave of labelled cells through a mitotic 'window'.

As with most techniques limitations are imposed by such factors as cell damage, sampling variation and intralesional variations. Hamilton and Berry [64] have suggested that thymidine tends to accumulate preferentially in well oxygenated cells and that tritiated uridine may give more representative results.

Autoradiographic methods could be used to predict human tumour responses to radiation and chemotherapy, especially where tumours are accessible to needle sampling – cervix uteri, head and neck, and lung.

A double labelling method using ^{3}H and ^{14}C-labelled thymidine has been introduced which allows assessment of the effects of cytotoxic drugs *in vivo* since it defines sub-populations of differently labelled cells in different phases and eliminates the need for synchronised cells [65].

11. Flow cytometry

This facility follows well-established principles to allow very rapid analysis of very large numbers of dispersed cells [66, 67].

The apparatus is shown diagramatically (Fig. 8). Fluid containing the discrete cells to be analysed is passed down a central tube with a small orifice. Cell-free fluid descends around this in a concentric chamber so that cells emerge one at a time in the centre of the stream. These individual cells can be assessed in various ways.

11.1. Cell impedance properties [68]

High frequency resistance and capacitance changes caused by passage of cells through the orifice can be measured and related to such properties as

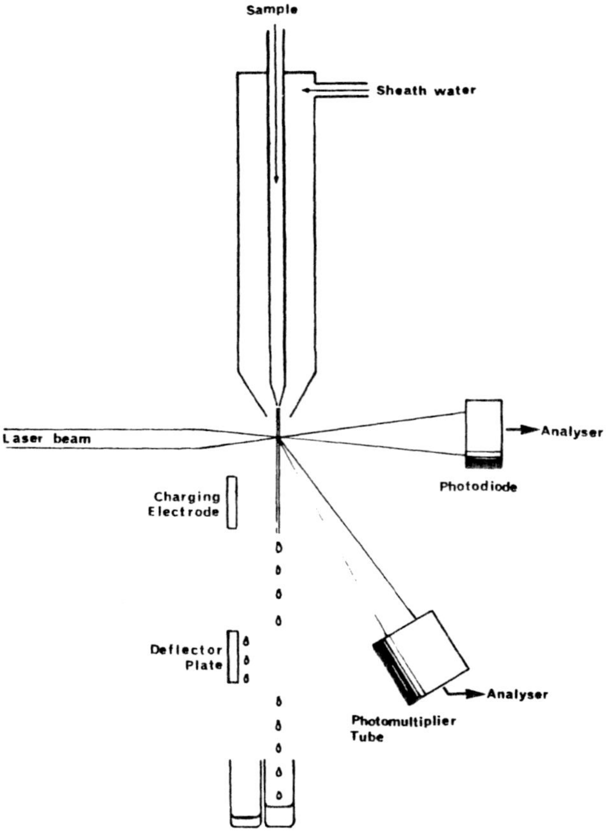

Figure 8. Diagramatic representation of elements used in flow cytometry.

cell volume, plasma membrane impedance and electrical sensitivity of the cell interior.

11.2. Multi-angle light scattering [69]

An argon laser beam focussed to give an elliptical cross-section at the intersection with the emerging cell stream gives rise to a scatter pattern when cells pass through it. A circular photo-diode can pick up the pattern which can be amplified and analysed by a linked computer system using an analog-to-digital convertor.

11.3. Fluorescence [70]

Several fluorescent dyes can be used, DNA is most commonly displayed but it is also possible to show RNA, protein and various enzymes. Acridine orange (AO) is versatile in giving green fluorescence with double-stranded nucleic acid (mostly DNA) and red fluorescence with single-stranded nucleic acid (mostly RNA). Acid denaturation preceding AO shows relatively high RNA in quiescent cells and relatively high DNA in cycling interphase cells [71]. This can be used to differentiate G_0 from G_1 cells and between G_2 and M cells. A second krypton laser beam is necessary for analysis of fluorescence of different wavelengths.

The fluorescent light pulses produced by stained cells passing through the laser beam(s) are received by photodetectors (photomultiplier tubes) placed at right angles to the beam. Signals are amplified, converted and recorded. If DNA is being measured, histograms can be prepared and these give a visual representation of the proportions of cells in different stages of the cycle. Data can be computer analysed to determine these proportions. Such information is much more quickly and easily obtained than from use of autoradiography and the labelling index. Correlation with results using autoradiography is good [72].

Therapeutic effects can be observed where the cell cycle is blocked and cells accumulate in an arrested phase. Alabaster *et al.* [73], have shown a possible alkylating effect of cyclophosphamide on guanine, using mithramycin which binds with guanine derivatives, and suggest that fluorescent probes may prove useful in detection of specific changes in macromolecular structure. They also indicate that measurement of fluorescence activity may afford a rapid assay of cell damage due to alkylation and may be especially useful with slow growing tumours.

Fluorescence activated cell sorters can sort the cells being discharged. The nozzle is made to vibrate rapidly so that the stream breaks up into droplets some distance below the nozzle. When a required characteristic is manifested by a cell passing through the laser beam, a charging electrode is made to charge the falling droplet with its contained cell. Charged droplets with their contained cells are deflected by a constantly charged deflection plate and can be collected for further examination. For instance, such cells can be tested for clonogenicty if the fluorescent dye is not significantly toxic. Certain benzimidazole dyes have been used successfully [74, 75]. This could be useful in examination of the effects of cytotoxic agents and in a selective study of the characteristics of cellular subpopulations.

Flow cytometry holds exciting prospects but the apparatus is elaborate and confined to research laboratories. While it will play a role in investigation of tumour biology, it is still constrained by many unresolved problems [76].

12. Summary and conclusions

The orthodox techniques of pathological examination, histology and cytology have been explored as the means of assessing response to treatment of neoplastic disease, but their incapacity to identify the vital, clonogenic, surviving fraction of such tumours has vitiated their value. Apart from ensuring that there is a response to irradiation in cervical tumours, microscopic examination is of limited relevance.

Numerous techniques have been applied to experimental tumours and these are particularly relevant to determination of tumour cell kinetics and clonogenicity. The value of these methods in assessment of human neoplasms is limited by various factors, especially the inaccessability of many tumours to repeated sampling, the problems of xenografting human tumours and poor plating efficiency of human tumour cells in artificial media. At present, it seems that these procedures offer most promise in examining effects of chemotherapeutic substances rather than in determining responsiveness of individual tumours.

References

1. Warren S, Meigs JV, Severance AO, Jaffe HL: The significance of the radiation reaction in carcinoma of the cervix uteri. Surg Gynecol Obstet 69:644–647, 1939.
2. Glucksman A: Preliminary observations on the quantitive examination of human biopsy material taken from irradiated carcinomata. Br J Radiol 14:187–198, 1941.
3. Glucksman A, Spear FG: The qualitive and quantitive histological examination of biopsy material from patients treated by radiation for carcinoma of the cervix uteri. Br J Radiol 18:313–322. 1945.
4. Glucksman A, Way S: On the choice of treatment of individual carcinoma of the cervic based on the analysis of serial biopsies. J Obstet Gynecol Br Emp 55:573–582, 1948.

5. Cherry CP, Glucksman A: The influence of systemic factors on the reaction to radiation treatment of the normal and malignant epithelium of the uterine cervix. Cancer 7:504–518, 1954.
6. Gusberg SB: A consideration of the problems of radiosensitivity in cancer of the cervix. Am J Obstet Gynecol 72:804–819, 1956.
7. Gusberg SB, Herman GG: Radio sensitivity testing of cervix cancer by the test dose technique. Am J Roentgen 87:60–68, 1962.
8. Dubrauszky V: Assessment of radiosensitivity of carcinoma of the cervix. J Obstet Gynecol Brit Cwlth 73:41–43, 1966.
9. Walter L, Harrison CV, Glucksman A, Cherry CP: Assessment of response of cervical cancer to irradiation by routine histological methods. Br Med J 1:1673–1675, 1964.
10. Thomlinson RH, Gray LH: The histological structure of some human lung cancers and the possible implications for radiotherapy. Br J Cancer 9:539–549, 1955.
11. Stenstrom KW, Vermund H, Mosser DG, Marvin JF: Effect of Roentgen irradiation on the tumour bed. 1. The inhibiting action of local pretransplantation Roentgen irradiation (1500 ra) on the growth of mouse mammary carcinoma. Radiation Res 2:180–191, 1954.
12. Hewitt HB, Blake ER: The growth of transplanted murine tumours in pre-irradiated sites. Br J Cancer 22:808–824, 1968.
13. Trott KR: Can tumour response be assessed from a biopsy? Br J Cancer 41 (Suppl IV):163–170, 1980.
14. Dische S, Bennett MH, Saunders MI, Anderson P: Tumour regression as a guide to prognosis. Br J Radiol 53:454–461, 1980.
15. Lokich JJ, Garnick MB, Legg M: Intralesional immune therapy. Oncology 36:236–241, 1979.
16. Kennedy PS, Smith B, McCracken JD: False positive Sternberg-Reed cells present in pericardial effusion. Arch Intern Med 138:1719–1720, 1978.
17. Fonts EA, Greenlaw RH, Rush BF, Rovin S: Verrucous squamous cell carcinoma of the oral cavity. Cancer 23:152–160, 1969.
18. Proffitt SD, Spooner TR, Kosek JC: Origin of undifferentiated neoplasm from verrucous epidermal carcinoma of oral cavity following irradiation. Cancer 26:389–393, 1970.
19. van Nostrand AWP, Olufsson J: Verrucous carcinoma of the larynx. Cancer 30:691–702, 1972.
20. Foulds L: The experimental study of tumour progression: a review. Cancer Res 14:327–339, 1954.
21. Lukes RJ, Collins RD: New approaches to classification of the lymphomata. Br J Cancer 31 (Suppl 11):1–28, 1975.
22. Everson TC, Cole WH: Spontaneous regression of cancer. Philadelphia: WB Saunders Co., 1966.
23. Rees GJG: Abscopal regression in lymphoma: a mechanism in common with total body irradiation. Clin Radiol 32:475–480, 1981.
24. Smith JA, Herr HW: Spontaneous regression of pulmonary metastases from transitional cell carcinoma. Câncer 46:1499–1502, 1980.
25. McCarthy WH, Shaw HM, Milton GW: Spontaneous regression of metastatic malignant melanoma. Clin Oncol 4:203–207, 1978.
26. Krutchick AN, Buzdar AU, Blumenschein GR, Lukeman JM: Spontaneous regression of breast carcinoma. Arch Intern Med 138:1734–1735, 1978.
27. Graham RM: The effect of radiation on vaginal cells in cervical carcinoma. Surg Gynecol Obstet 84:153–165, 1947.
28. Graham RM, Graham JB: A cellular index of sensitivity to ionising radiation: The sensitisation response. Cancer 6:215–223, 1953.
29. Graham RM, Graham JB: Cytological prognosis in cancer of the uterine cervix treated radiologically. Cancer 8:59–70, 1955.

30. Graham RM: Cytologic prognosis in cancer of cervix. Am J Obstet Gynecol 79:700–708, 1960.
31. Graham RM, Graham JB: Cytologic prognosis in cancer of the cervix; two year survival rates in a randomised series. Am J Roentgen 87:56–59, 1962.
32. Agnew AM, Fidler HK, Boyes DA: Evaluation of radiation response. Am J Obstet Gynecol 79:698–699. 1960.
33. Rubio CA, Hertzberg O, Kottmeier H-L, Olsson E, Zejicek J: Sensitisation and radiation response in cases with carcinoma of the uterine cervix. Acta Radiologica (Therapy) 3:241–268, 1965.
34. Wachtel E: A simple cytological test for cancer cure. Br Med J 1:20–22, 1958.
35. Jones HW, Goldberg B, Davis HJ, Burns BC Jr: Cellular changes in vaginal and buccal smears after radiation. An index of the radiocurability of carcinoma of the cervix. Am J Obstet Gynecol 78:1083–1100, 1959.
36. Marshall MJ, Neal FE, Goldberg DM: Effect of radiotherapy upon enzymes of the glycolytic and related pathways in human uterine cancer. Br J Cancer 39, 90–95, 1979.
37. Taper HS, Deckers Co, Deckers Passau LO: Increase in nuclease activity as a possible means for detecting tumour cell sensitivity to anticancer agents. Cancer 47:523–529, 1981.
38. De Brabander MJ, Van de Veire RML, Aerts FEM, Borgess M, Janssen PAJ: The effects of methyl [5-(2-thienylcarbanyl)-1H-benzimidazol-2-yl] carbamate (R 17934; NSC 238159), a new synthetic antitumoural drug interfering with microtubules, on mammalian cells cultured *in-vitro*. Cancer Res 36:905–916, 1976.
39. Hill RP: An appraisal of *in-vivo* assays of excised tumours. Br J Cancer 41 (Suppl IV):230–239, 1980.
40. Hewitt HB, Wilson CW: A survival curve for mammalian leukaemia cells irradiated *in-vivo*, (Indications for the treatment of mouse leukaemia by whole body irradiation). Br J Cancer 13:69–75, 1959.
41. Hewitt HB, Chan D P-S, Blacke ER: Survival curves for clonogenic cells of a murine keratinising squamous carcinoma irradiated *in-vivo* under hypoxic conditions. Int J Radiat Biol 12:535–549, 1967.
42. Clifton KH, Draper NR: Survival curves of solid transplantable tumour cells irradiated *in-vivo*: a method of determination and statistical evaluation: comparison of cell survival and ^{32}P uptake into DNA. Int J Radiat Biol 7:515–535, 1963.
43. Begg AC: Analysis of growth delay data: Potential pitfalls. Br J Cancer 41 (Suppl IV):93–97, 1980.
44. Hill RP, Bush RS: A lung colony assay to determine the radiosensitivity of the cells in a solid tumour. Int J Radiat Biol 15:435–444, 1969.
45. Revesz L: Effect of tumour cells killed by X-rays upon the growth of admixed viable cells. Nature 178:1391–1392, 1956.
46. Castro JE: Human tumours grown in mice. Nature (New Biol) 239:83–84, 1972.
47. Selby PJ, Thomas JM, Monaghan P, Sloane J, Peckham MJ: Human tumour xenografts established and serially transplanted in mice immunologically deprived by thymectomy, cytosine arabinoside and whole body irradiation. Br J Cancer 41:52–61, 1980.
48. Shorthouse AJ, Smyth JF, Steel GG, Ellison M, Mills J, Peckham MJ: The human tumour xenograft – a valid model in experimental chemotherapy. Br J Surg 67:715–722, 1980.
49. Bailey MJ, Gazet J-C, Peckham MJ: Human breast-cancer xenografts in immune suppressed mice. Br J Cancer 42:524–529, 1980.
50. Rygaard J, Povlsen CO: Heterotransplantation of a human malignant tumour to 'nude' mice. Acta Path Microbiol Scand 77:758–760, 1969.
51. Kyriazis AK, Kyriazis AP: Preferential sites of growth of human tumours in nude mice following subcutaneous transplantation. Cancer Res 40:4509–4511, 1980.

52. Davies G, Duke D, Grant AG, Kelly SA, Hermon-Taylor J: Growth of human digestive tumour xenografts in athymic nude rats. Br J Cancer 43:53–58, 1981.
53. Courtenay VD, Smith IE, Peckham MJ, Steel GG: *In-vitro* and *in-vivo* radiosensitivity of human tumour cells obtained from a pancreatic carcinoma xenograft. Nature 263:771–772, 1976.
54. Courtenay VD, Mills J: An *in-vitro* colony assay for human tumours grown in immune suppressed mice and treated *in-vivo* with cytotoxic agents. Br J Cancer 37:261–268, 1978.
55. Ozols RF, Wilson JKV, Grotzinger KR, Young RC: Cloning of human ovarian cancer cells in soft agar from malignant effusions and peritoneal washings. Cancer Res 40:2743–2747, 1980.
56. Ozols RF, Wilson JKV, Weltz MD: Inhibition of human ovarian cancer colony formation by Adriamycin and its major metabolites. Cancer Res 40:4109–4112, 1980.
57. Barendsen GW: Analysis of tumour responses by excision and *in-vitro* assay of cellular clonogenic capacity. Br J Cancer 41 (Suppl IV):209–216, 1980.
58. Sutherland RM, Durand RE: Hypoxic cells in an *in-vitro* tumour model. Int J Radiat Biol 23:235–246, 1973.
59. Olive PL: Different sensitivity to cytotoxic agents of internal and external cells of spheroids composed of thioguanine-resistant and sensitive cells. Br J Cancer 43:85–92, 1981.
60. Yanagita T, Herman GG, Gusberg SB: Autoradiographic studies in cervical cancer before and after a test dose of irradiation. Am J Obstet Gynecol 95:1051–1058, 1966.
61. Bresciani F, Paoluzi R, Benassi M, Nervi C, Casale C, Ziporo E: Cell kinetics and growth of squamous cell carcinomas in man. Cancer Res 34:2405–2415, 1974.
62. Strauss MJ, Morgan RE: Cell cycle parameters in human solid tumours. Cancer 40:1453–1461, 1977.
63. Nervi C, Badaracco G, Morelli M, Starace G: Cytokinetic evaluation in human head and neck cancer by autoradiography and DNA cytofluorimetry. Cancer 46:452–459, 1980.
64. Hamilton E, Berry RJ: *In-situ* measures of tumour cell proliferation and their relation to models of tumour growth. Br J Cancer 41 (Suppl IV):98, 1980.
65. Schultze B: Double labelling autoradiography and cell kinetic studies with ^{3}H- and ^{14}C-thymidine. J Histochem Cytochem Suppl 29:109–116, 1981.
66. Steinkamp JA, Fulwyler MJ, Coulter JR, Hiebert RD, Horney JL, Mullaney PF: A new multiparameter separator for microscopic particles and biological cells. Rev Sci Instrum 44:1301–1310, 1973.
67. Watson JV: Identification of different cell types and their separation using flow cytometric systems. In: Cancer assessment and monitoring, Symington T, Williams AE, McVie JG (eds). Edinburgh: Churchill Livingstone, 1980, pp 77–95.
68. Hoffman RA, Britt WB: Flow-system measurement of cell impedance properties. J Histochem Cytochem 27:234–240, 1979.
69. Salzman GC, Crowell JM, Goad CA, Hansen KM, Hiebert RD, La Bauve PM, Martin JC, Ingram ML, Mullaney PF: A flow system multiangle light-scattering instrument for cell characterisation. Clin Chem 21:1297–1304, 1975.
70. Crissman HA, Oka MS, Steinkamp JA: Rapid staining methods for analysis of deoxyribonucleic acid and protein in mammalian cells. J Histochem Cytochem 24:64–71, 1976.
71. Darzynkiewicz Z, Traganos F, Andreef M, Sharpless T, Melamed MR: Different sensitivity of chromatin to acid denaturation in quiescent and cycling cells as revealed by flow cytometry. J Histochem Cytochem 27:478–485, 1979.
72. Linden WA, Köllerman M, König K: Flow cytometric and autoradiographic studies of human kidney carcinomas surgically removed after pre-irradiation. Br J Cancer 41 (Suppl IV):177–180, 1980.
73. Alabaster O, Magrath IT, Habbersett MC, Herman CJ: Effects of cyclophosphamide on the mithramycin – DNA fluorescence of human lymphoma cells: a possible result of guanine alkylation. J Histochem Cytochem 27:500–504, 1979.

74. Arndt-Jovin DJ, Jovin TM: Analysis and sorting of living cells according to deoxyribonucleic acid content. J Histochem Cytochem 25:585–589, 1977.
75. Pallavicini MG, La Lande ME, Miller RG, Hill RP: Cell cycle distribution of chronically hypoxic cells and determination of the clonogenic potential of cells accumulated in G_2 and M phases after irradiation of a solid tumour *in-vivo.* Cancer Res 39:1891–1897, 1979.
76. Raju MR, Johnson TS, Tokita N, Gillette EL: Flow cytometric applications to tumour biology: prospects and pitfalls. Br J Cancer 41 (Suppl IV):171–176, 1980.

8. Chromosomal Changes

A. M. POTTER

1. Introduction

Technical improvements over the last thirty years have allowed cytogeneticists to examine the chromosome complements of a large variety of cancers. This work has shown that most, but not all, cancers exhibit chromosome abnormalities. Malignant tissue may demonstrate a change from the normal diploid number as a result of loss or gain of chromosomes through errors in cell division, or from structurally altered 'marker' chromosomes resulting from chromosome breakage and reunion. Frequently both types of abnormality are present. These chromosome changes can be induced by physical agents, particularly ionising radiation, or by a wide range of chemical substances. Some may act directly on the chromosome to produce lesions whilst others, by inhibiting the normal cell repair mechanism, allow the accumulation of spontaneously occurring chromosome breaks and interchanges. Changes in the chromosome number can occur when interference with the mitotic mechanisms of the cell causes mis-segregation producing loss or gain of a particular chromosome (aneuploidy) or duplication of the diploid set of chromosomes (polyploidy). These anomalies are confined to malignant tissue, and differ in this respect from congenital chromosome abnormalities where the aberrant cells are distributed throughout the body. These latter abnormalities are, of course, associated with developmental congenital malformations.

2. Historical background

The significance of chromosome changes in cancer has been a matter of controversy from the beginning of the present century. Workers at that time were able to observe abnormal mitoses which would give rise to cells with abnormal chromosome numbers, although direct examination of the karyotype of cancer cells was not possible until the early 1950s. It was the observation of aberrant mitoses by a number of scientists that led Theodore Boveri, during his study of tripolar cell division in starfish, to publish a theory linking abnormal chromosome complements to cancer.

He suggested that any mechanism producing an alteration in chromosome

Hancock, B. W. (ed.), Assessment of Tumour Response.
 ISBN 90-247-2712-X.
Printed in The Netherlands.

number could result in cells with an excess of chromosomes containing 'growth promoting factors' and loss of chromosomes containing 'growth inhibiting factors'. Such cells would gain a selective advantage over normal cells by virtue of their growth potential, and Boveri proposed in his Chromosome Theory of Cancer [1] that cancers might develop in this manner. This was the first attempt to suggest a causal relationship between chromosome abnormality and malignant growth but, at the time of its publication, Boveri's theory proved of little interest to cancer workers.

Confirmation that many cancer cells are chromosomally abnormal was first provided by Winge [2] in plant tumours and it was Winge who first introduced the concept that tumours might be composed of cells with a range of chromosome abnormalities. This work was continued with the pioneer studies on experimental tumours, including the analysis of the Yoshida Rat Sarcoma [3] and the studies on free cell ascites tumours [4].

2.1. Stem line concept

Subsequently, a large number of solid tumours in humans have been analysed. The first study by Makino *et al.* [7] was of nineteen solid human tumours at seven different sites and demonstrated modal numbers between 53 and 84. Spriggs *et al.* [6], studying primary tumours of the cervix, lung and brain, showed that a variety of aberrations were often present within the same tumour. The finding of cells with the same abnormal chromosome suggested these were derived from a single cell and hence represented a clone. We now know that large variations in karyotype exist from tumour to tumour and that there are no simple chromosome changes common to all tumours.

The first suitable material in which heterogeneity of the tumour could be accurately analysed were the ascites tumours investigated by Levan and Hauschka [4]. This work has shown that, within the tumour, cells with differing chromosome numbers coexist, with the modal number occurring in the dominant clone. When cells with the modal number also have the same chromosome complement, this would suggest that they are derived from a common ancestor. These cells are designated the stemline of the tumour. Makino [5] put forward the theory that the heterogeneous structure of tumours enhances their progression, and that the variety of cell lines with different karyotypes represents a pool which will provide the basis for adaptation to changes in the environment. Shifts in the cancer stemline or the appearance of new variants in the chromosome complement could therefore be viewed as part of the adaptive changes occurring during the development of the cancer.

3. Chromosome changes in leukaemia

Most solid tumours, unfortunately, do not provide large numbers of analysable metaphases because technical difficulties are encountered when processing biopsied material. A further problem is that the tissue is usually obtained from established tumours. These tumours are difficult to analyse because of the complexity of the karyotype abnormalities and rarely demonstrate further chromosome changes, except of a comparatively minor nature.

While some chromosomal responses are well illustrated in the study of experimental tumours, the leukaemias provide far more suitable material for the cytogeneticist to observe chromosome evolution in a naturally occurring cancer in man.

One form of leukaemia which has proved particularly useful in demonstrating the appearance of abnormal clones is chronic myeloid leukaemia (CML). This disease has been shown to be characterised by a specific chromosome aberration known as the Philadelphia chromosome (Ph′). During the course of CML a benign phase lasting an average of three years transforms into an acute phase accompanied by a series of well-documented chromosome changes.

Here, as in many other myeloid leukaemias, the chromosome aberrations are relatively simple and the sequence of chromosome changes can usually be confidently derived. The events can be easily followed as sampling of blood and marrow are a matter of routine during treatment. Furthermore, because the aberrations observed are confined to one or two chromosomes, there is the opportunity to monitor the role of specific chromosome markers in the evolution of the disease.

3.1. Chromosome abnormalities and prognosis

It has been suggested that the heterogeneous cell population of cancers is an aid to their progression. The demonstration of cells with an abnormal chromosome constitution or the observation of the emergence of a new clone may therefore be significant to prognosis. Some characteristic changes in cancer have been related to chromosome changes. Resistance to a variety of drugs has been studied using for the most part experimental tumours, and this resistance has frequently, but not always, been associated with the appearance of new chromosome anomalies. Hauschka [8] reported that amethopterin-resistant sub-lines of Erlich ascites not only had a different modal number but contained two characteristic chromosome markers. A similar situation has been observed in radiation-resistant tumours and when studying the ability to transplant tumours. The acquisition of these characters has been found frequently to be accompanied by the emergence of a new modal cell line. For example, Hauschka and Levan [9] established a close relationship between chromosome constitution and the antigenic differentiation needed for the successful grafting of a tumour to a new host. These changes are frequently dependent on the evolution of an abnormal karyotype and successful transplantation has been found to increase with a rise in the chromosome number.

3.1.1. Acute leukaemias. In both acute lymphoblastic leukaemia (ALL) and acute non-lymphoblastic leukaemia (ANLL), the marrow karyotype has been reported to be chromosomally abnormal in approximately 50% of cases. The further evolution of the karyotype, when it occurs, does not appear to be of particular clinical significance. Thus those individuals with a normal complement at diagnosis usually fail to evolve abnormal clones, even when long survivors are studied. Whang-Peng *et al.* [10] found that in those cases with abnormal chromosomes successful chemotherapy usually results in a reversion to a normal karyotype, although the original abnormal clone is likely to reappear or be replaced by a new clone when the patient relapses. This phenomenon is more frequently observed in cases of ALL, where remissions are more readily induced.

Although in this instance the presence or absence of chromosome changes appears to be related to the clinical phase of the disease, a number of researchers have studied median survival times of cases of acute leukaemia in relation to their karyotype. Sakurai and Sandberg [11] divided a series of patients with acute myeloid leukaemia (AML) into three groups: those with normal karyotypes (NN), those with abnormal karyotypes (AA) and those with both types (AN). These authors reported that the median life spans of AA cases, either from the time of diagnosis or from when treatment was begun, were significantly shorter than AN cases, and that NN cases appear to have the longest survival time. The same finding may be true for ALL where Whang-Peng [10] found longer NN survival times when compared with AA patients although these findings have not yet been confirmed. One problem in assessing this data, particularly in NN patients, is the inability of cytogeneticists to distinguish whether chromosomally normal cells include of a mixture of non-leukaemic and leukaemic cells.

Sakurai and Sandberg [11] suggest that the important factor in these findings is the presence of normal diploid cells rather than the chromosome constitution of the AA patients. Although no consistent chromosome markers have been identified in ALL, a number of non-random chromosome abnormalities are associated with ANLL patients, the commonest of these being a rearrangement between chromosomes 8 and 21 (8/21 translocation) and an extra chromosome 8 (trisomy 8).

It has not as yet been possible to demonstrate whether the appearance of a

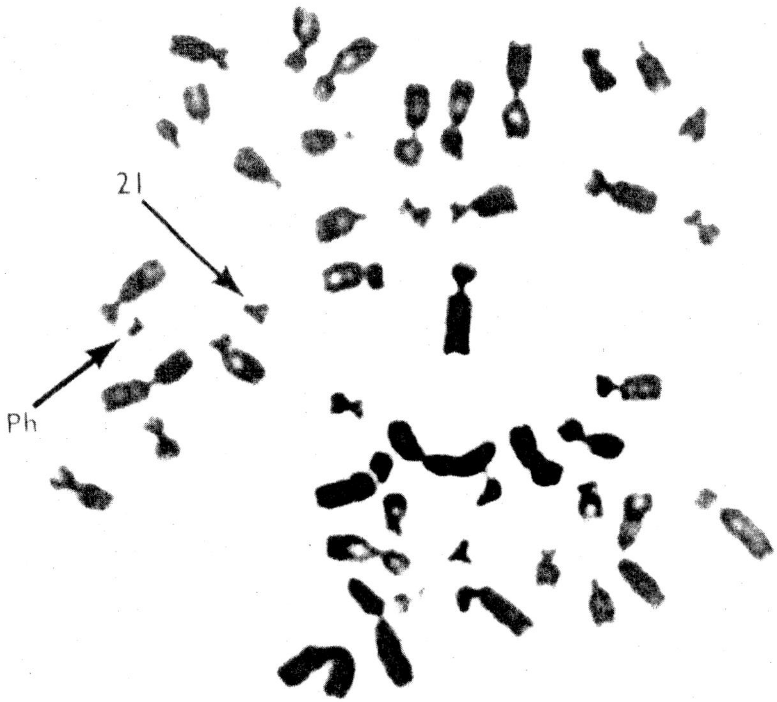

Figure 1. Non-banded metaphase with Philadelphia chromosome (Ph^1) arrowed, and normal 'G-group' chromosome (21) for comparison.

particular chromosome alters the prognosis. Bloomfield *et al.* [12] have suggested that the presence of a Philadelphia chromosome in both AML and ALL significantly shortens survival times when compared with other AA cases. Although this has not been confirmed by some other reports, differences in both chemotherapy and diagnostic criteria between different centres may make comparison of such data invalid.

3.1.2. Chronic myeloid leukaemia. In 90% of patients in whom chronic myeloid leukaemia (CML) has been diagnosed, a small abnormal chromosome known as the Philadelphia chromosome (Ph^1) can be observed in the marrow cells. This marker is confined to the granulocytes, erythrocytes and megakaryocytes, and those cases where the Ph^1 cannot be demcnstrated probably constitute a distinct and separate disease variant (Fig. 1).

The Ph^1 was first described by Nowell and Hungerford in 1960 [13], and this finding of a specific chromosome marker with such consistency at the onset of a malignant disease created an upsurge of interest in chromosome markers in cancer. In this case the Ph^1 may represent a chromosome change which is directly related to the initiation of the disease process. Rowley [14] demonstrated that the Ph^1 is produced by a segment of long arm chromo-

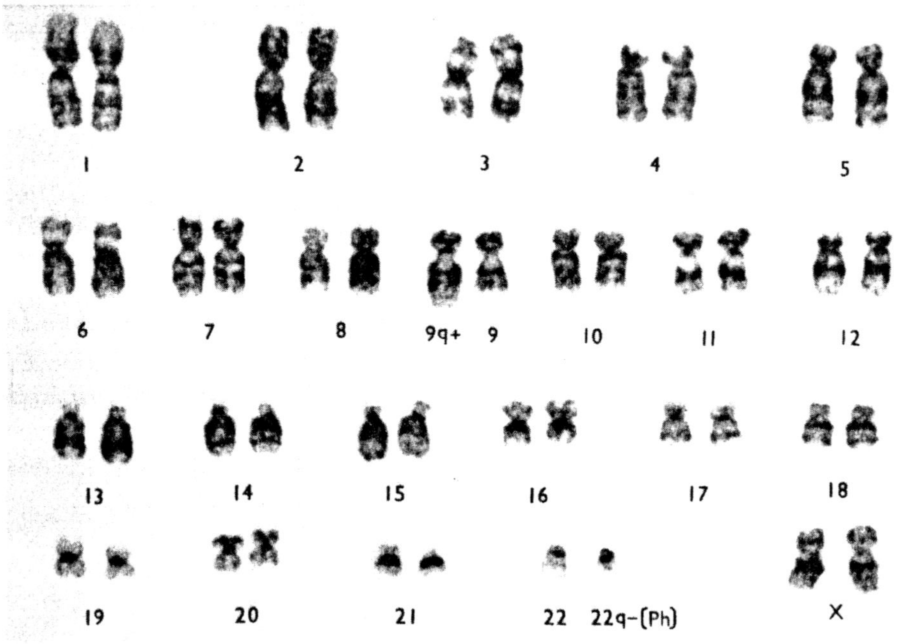

Figure 2. Karyotype of banded cell showing the Philadelphia chromosome to be a 9/22 translocation.

some 22 becoming repositioned (translocated) onto the long arm of a 9 chromosome (Fig 2). Although this is the most common translocation, the long arm segment from the 22 chromosome can be translocated onto other chromosomes. Although Sonta and Sandberg [15] did not detect any prognostic significance in Ph^1 chromosome derived from non 9/22 rearrangements, Potter *et al.* [16] reported that these unusual rearrangements were associated with both older and short-surviving patients. Balanced translocations, in which there has been no loss or gain of genetic material, do not usually give rise to detectable clinical changes. These changes are due to the new association within the chromosome of structural heterochromatic regions with genetically active euchromatic regions effecting transcription and is known as the position effect. It may therefore be that any prognostic differences seen in these cases represents different expressions of a position effect.

Not all CML cases present at the time of diagnosis with the Ph^1 as the sole chromosome aberration and it is important to establish the karyotype at this time in order to distinguish the primary chromosome changes from subsequent chromosome evolution. The most common types of aberration appearing at the time the Ph^1 is formed are balanced translocations, and the loss of a Y chromosome in male patients. Although Sakurai and Sandberg [17] suggested that the latter aberration might enhance survival times, the role of this missing Y in CML remains unresolved; neither type of aberration has as yet been shown to contribute to the evolution of the disease.

A small number of cases demonstrate a mixture of chromosomally normal cells and Ph+ cells. These mosaics may represent an early and transient stage of the disease in which non-leukaemic cells are still detectable in marrow analyses. Those patients in which this mosaicism persists show a tendency to prolonged survival [18] and within this group are patients who exhibit an increased sensitivity to chemotherapy [19]. This situation may be analogous to that seen in acute leukaemia and reflect the advantage of normal cells co-existing with leukaemic clones. Such observations have suggested that a more radical treatment of CML in the chronic phase aimed at the elimination of the Ph^1 clone might improve survival prospects.

A number of cancers are believed to be derived from a single cell. Evidence for this view rests mainly on a study of individuals whose normal tissues are made up of a mixture of more than one cell type. Such diversity can be observed in cases which are heterozygous for an X-linked marker or in those which have congenital chromosome mosaicism. In CML Fialkow *et al.* [20 studied heterozygotes for the sex linked enzyme glucose-6-dehydrogenase and found, in seven cases, only one form of the isoenzyme to be present in the Ph^1 cells.

Confirmation of this evidence was presented by Fitzgerald *et al.* [21] who reported a somatic mosaic 46,XY/47,XXY individual in whom the Ph^1 was only present in the 46,XY cell line. However, in a contradictory report by Tough *et al.* [22], a similar 46,XY/47,XXY mosaic was found to have a Ph^1

Table 1. Dates of reviews demonstrating stages of chromosome evolution in Case I

Days from diagnosis	Karyotype	Percentage
1	46, XY,Ph^1	100%
828	46, XY, Ph^1	100%
1017	46, XY, Ph^1 46, XY, Phq+	82% 18%
1192	46, XY, Ph^1 46, XY, Phq+	15% 85%
1353	46, XY, Ph^1 46, XY, Phq+ 48, Ph^1, +Ph^1, +8	4% 74% 22%
1381	46, XY, Ph^1 49, XY, Ph^1, Ph^1, +8, +mar	7% 93%
1409	49, XY,Ph^1, Ph^1, +8, +mar	100%

chromosome present in both cell lines. Although the findings in CML are not conclusive, the weight of evidence in many other leukaemias supports the monoclonal origin of these diseases.

Nevertheless, new abnormal clones do occasionally appear in the benign phase of the disease which do not herald any change in the disease status. In our experience, these clones rarely grow at the expense of the original Ph^1 cell line and often are not observed in later samples. In some cases these clones are able to slowly dominate the marrow and this development is a more significant signal of an acceleration in the disease. Case I (Table 1) and Case II (Table 2) illustrate this form of chromosome evolution.

Table 2. Dates of reviews demonstrating stages of chromosome evolution in Case II

Days from diagnosis	Karyotype	Percentage
1	46, XY, Ph^1	100%
512	46, XY, Ph^1 45, X, Ph^1	30% 70%
789	45, X, Ph^1	100%
1004	45, X, Ph^1 46, X, Ph^1, Ph^1	20% 80%
1130	45, X, Ph^1 46, X, Ph^1, Ph^1	7% 93%
1279	45, X, Ph^1, −17, i(17q) 46, X, Ph^1, Ph^1	50% 50%
1333	45, X, Ph^1, −17, i(17q)	100%

Case I. A 37-year-old man was monitored during the benign phase. For the first 30 months only a single 46,XY,Ph^1 cell line was observed. A new clone with an extra unidentified segment translocated onto the Ph^1 was then seen and over the next 12 months the proportion of this new clone increased from 18% to 94% of the cells. Apart from a fall in the haemoglobin levels the patient remained well during this period. However, after 12 months a third clone evolved with 48 chromosomes but, as the abnormal Phq+ was not observed, this must have been derived from the 46,XY,Ph^1 cell line. During the following month the third cell line increased and evolved further and at this time acute transformation was diagnosed.

Case II. A 48-year-old man at diagnosis had two cell lines, 46,XY,Ph^1/45,X,Ph^1. After six months all cells seen were without the Y chromosome and for a further 17 months the patient continued in the benign phase with this karyotype until a new clone with 2Ph^1's was detected. This new line, originally in only 20% of cells, eventually appeared

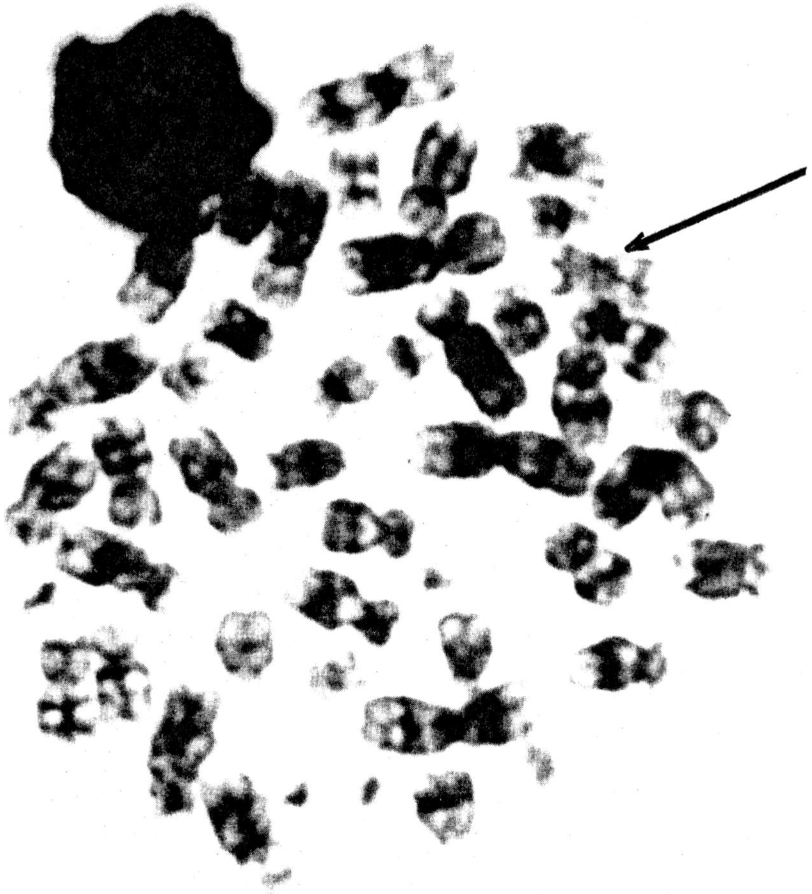

Figure 3. Metaphase from CML to blast transformation with isochromosome long arm 17 arrowed, resulting in duplication of the long arm of chromosome 17 and loss of the short arm.

in 97% of cells. Although during this time the white blood count started to rise and the patient became unwell, transformation did not occur until a further cell line with an abnormal chromosome 17 (isochromosome long arm 17) appeared. Within two months of the emergence of this new clone the patient had become resistant to Busulphan and transformed (Fig. 3).

Between 80 and 90% of marrows from patients with CML at blast transformation have evolved new chromosome aberrations. The appearance of these new clones can be detected 2 to 6 months prior to transformation. In contrast to those clones seen during the benign phase, the Ph^1 cell line is rapidly overtaken by those clones as demonstrated in the above examples. Although more radical drug regimes are adopted during the acute phase, remissions are rarely obtained, but in the few cases when this occurs, the

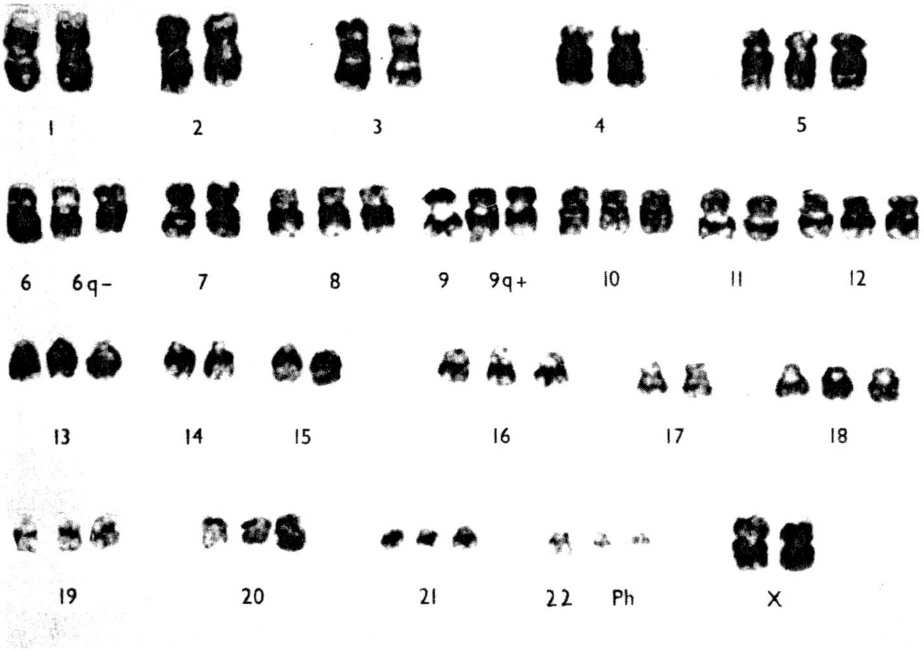

Figure 4. Karyotype from a transformed Ph[1] CML patient with 59 chromosomes present.

karyotype reverts to the original Ph[1] cell line. Otherwise further chromosome evolution is frequently observed as seen in Case III (Table 3).

Table 3. Dates if reviews demonstrating stages of chromosome evolution in Case III

Days from diagnosis	Karyotype	Percentage
1	46, XY,Ph[1]	70%
	46, XY, N.A.D.	30%
343	46, XY, Ph[1]	100%
656	46, XY, Ph[1]	87%
	47, XY, Ph[1], −17, i(17q)	13%
731	46, XY, Ph[1], −17, +i(17q)	11%
	47, XY, Ph[1], −17, +i(17q), +19	12%
	48, XY, Ph[1], −17, +i(17q), +8, +19	77%

Case III. A 54-year-old man presented at diagnosis with two cell lines, 46,XY/46,XY,Ph[1]. However, chromosome analysis a year later failed to detect any normal cells. The patient remained in the benign phase for three years when an i(17q) chromosome appeared in 13% of cells.

Two months later the patient had transformed and all the cells now had an i(17q) present, together with a further chromosome abnormality. A subsequent sample one month later showed a further evolution of this clone with three derivative cell lines now present.

The chromosome abnormalities seen at transformation have been shown by a number of workers to be non-random [14, 23]. These abnormalities are listed in Table 4 and occur either together with random abnormalities or in combination with each other. Mitelman *et al.* [24] has suggested that these markers appear in a stepwise series in which the duplication of the chromosomes involved takes place in a set sequence. Certainly some combinations of chromosome abnormalities, for example a second Ph[1] together with isochromosome long arm 17, never appear. Although the significance of this is not understood it could be explained by certain chromosome changes triggering the generation of new aberrations. Alternatively, if these changes are modifying the growth and survival of the cells in which they are found, some specific combinations may do so to the extent that these cells are no longer capable of survival. Thus, the presence of extra markers may not have a simply additive effect.

Prigogina *et al.* [25] reported that from a series of 24 cases those who transformed without chromosome changes other than a Ph[1] survived longer and were more likely to have remissions when compared with patients with additional chromosome changes. Whilst our own data would tend to confirm this finding, Sonta and Sandberg [26] failed to detect any differences in the survival times of patients whether or not additional abnormalities had been observed at transformation. Such comparisons are more difficult when any attempt is made to quantify the effect of a particular chromosome marker. Many patients, at transformation, demonstrate a heterogeneous population of cells which undergo further evolution throughout the acute phase, and it is evident that large numbers of cases must be studied in order to establish this type of correlation.

Table 4. Some marker chromosomes specifically associated with particular malignancies

Chromosome abnormality		Type of malignancy
9/22	Balanced translocation	Chronic myeloid leukaemia (CML)
8/14	Balanced translocation	Burkitt's lymphoma
i(17q)	Isochromosome 17	Blast phase CML
20q–	Deleted chromosome 20	Polycythaemia vera
15/17	Balanced translocation	Promyelocytic leukaemia
Trisomy 8	Extra chromosome 8	AML and myeloproliferative disorders
5q–	Deleted chromosome 5	Refractory anaemia
Monosomy 22	Missing chromosome 22	Meningiomas

4. The role of specific chromosome markers in cancer (see Table 4)

Boveri's theory, suggesting that malignancy might be a product of changes from the normal diploid karyotype, presupposes that cancer cells would possess non-random chromosome abnormalities and that specific chromosomes or parts of chromosomes could be important in stem line concept and be sensitive to the same laws apparent in experimental tumours. However, some chromosome changes are certainly random although some of these will certainly also represent malignant changes.

Mitelman and Levan [27] have suggested that chromosome aberrations might be of two types. The first, a primary change involving small structural changes in the chromosome and including undetectable mutations at the gene level, would be associated with the primary events of carcinogenesis. Other secondary chromosome aberrations may act to complement or interact with the primary lesion. Such secondary changes could be generated randomly, in which case the emergence of dominant cell lines would be the result of selection for those cells in which the particular aberration confers some advantage in terms of growth or survival. Alternatively, triggered in some way by the primary lesion, there may be selective generation of specific chromosome abnormalities which directly, or by the induction of further changes, produce an enhanced growth potential in the cells which carry them.

5. Chromosome abnormalities arising due to treatment

Although a variety of leukaemias, and in particular the acute leukaemias, demonstrate chromosome abnormalities appearing prior to therapy, many malignancies are treated with agents that are themselves mutagenic. Since Muller [28] first demonstrated the mutagenic effects of X-rays on Drosophilia, extensive data has been collected on the ability of ionising radiation to induce chromosome aberrations. Much of this work has been available from the study of victims of the atomic bombing in Japan in 1945 [29]. Increase in chromosomal damage observed in lymphocytes in these cases is related to the calculated exposure to ionising radiation, and is accompanied by an increased incidence of leukaemias and other cancers. Treatment with X-rays, for instance for ankylosing spondylitis, has also led to an increased incidence of malignancies. A similar situation has been reported for a variety of chemical agents. Benzene has been shown to cause cancer and to induce increased chromosome damage. Many of the drugs used for the treatment of leukaemias, including folic acid inhibitors (e.g. methotrexate) and cytostatic drugs (e.g. actinomycin and busulphan), can cause chromosome breaks. Such treatment may, therefore, either initiate or enhance the appearance of chromosomally abnormal clones found in treated patients. Such a situation is exemplified in the case of Polycythaemia rubra vera (PRV).

PRV is a chronic myeloproliferative disease in which there is hyperplasia of all bone marrow elements. Although the course of the disease is variable, between 10 and 15% of cases undergo a malignant transformation with changes typical of acute myeloblastic leukaemia. Testa [30], in a review of the literature, reported that 13% of untreated cases have abnormal clones present, whereas 38% of treated cases show abnormal clones. When treated cases, which have developed leukaemia, are studied, 82% are found to have abnormal clones.

The pattern of chromosome abnormalities in PRV is non-random. The cell lines with extra chromosomes from pairs 8 and 9 are seen mainly in patients who have not undergone treatment. However, structural rearrange-

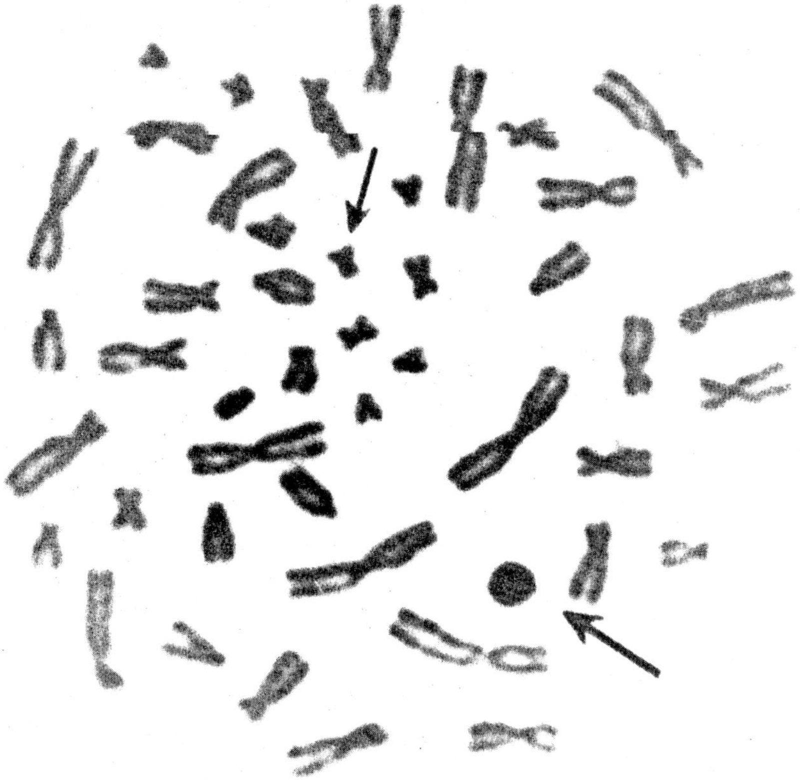

Figure 5. Cell from patient with transforming P.R.V. with deleted chromosome 20 arrowed. A further ring present is also arrowed.

ments involving chromosome No. 1 and No. 20 are frequently associated with patients treated with 32p or chemical agents.

Chromosome No. 20 with a segment lost from the long arm is the most common abnormality found in up to 30% of chromosomally abnormal PRV cases, and was originally thought to be specifically associated with 32P treatment. However, it has now been shown that some untreated cases may have this abnormality. Unlike CML the observation of these abnormal clones is not a clear indication of an imminent leukaemic transformation, although such patients usually have a poorer prognosis than those with normal karyotypes.

In normal lymphocytes Honeycombe [31] has reported non-random distribution of breaks induced by busulphan. However, the sites of breakage do not appear to correspond to the breakpoints producing the chromosome rearrangements characteristic of myeloid leukaemia. Non-random break sites have also been reported using mitomycin C [32] and chlorambucil [33].

These results suggest that treatment with mutagenic drugs may be a contributory factor in the production of abnormal clones. Rowley [34] has suggested that in the case of PRV there may be a fragile site on the long arm of chromosome No. 20 which is particularly susceptible to the action of mutagenic types of therapy and which provides a clone with a proliferative advantage. Such a site would not, therefore, be present in the lymphocytes from healthy individuals.

6. Significance of chromosome changes

The problem of the significance of chromosome changes in cancer remains unresolved despite the wealth of new information on karyotype changes now available. Much of the data reported concerns the myeloid leukaemias where new clones have been shown to develop during the course of the disease and where there is some evidence that the finding of chromosome abnormality might effect prognosis.

Chromosome changes present at the time the disease is diagnosed may have a direct involvement in the causation of the disease. Although it is not known whether the chromosome changes associated with the formation of the Ph′ are directly responsible for CML, there is a strong case for this because of the consistency of the Ph′ in the early stages of the disease. Recent studies on Burkitt's lymphoma have revealed a similar early association between this disease and an 8/14 translocation. It is possible that technical improvements giving high resolution of chromosomes may reveal further previously undetected chromosome changes of this type.

Most of the chromosomally abnormal clones seen in cancer cells are secondary events and represent the evolution of the stem line. Whatever factors might be responsible for the initiation of the disease, there is no reason to believe that the acquisition of malignancy should not be a continuing process and that the development of new karyotypic combinations might play a part in freeing these cells from the normal restraints on uncontrolled growth. The stepwise evolution of chromosome change demonstrated in CML, associated with new and more agressive growth, argues that these changes are part of the malignant changes observed rather than merely accidental byproducts of another process.

A second problem is how the non-random chromosome changes arise. One possibility is that agents capable of disrupting the chromosomes generate a series of random chromosome abnormalities and from these, mutations capable of promoting malignant growth would be selected. Certain aberrations might be advantageous to growth only in specific tissue and this would explain the finding of consistent chromosome markers restricted to particular leukaemic sub-groups.

A second explanation of the appearance of non-random chromosome changes depends on the ability of carcinogens to produce lesions at specific chromosome sites. Such a view is supported by reports that some chromosome aberrations have a specific geographical distribution [27] and that certain chemically-induced cancers have been shown to have markers specific for the carcinogenic agent used rather than the site of the tumour [35]. Although there is no reason to believe that these two possible ways of generating abnormal chromosomes are mutually exclusive, it is important to determine the derivation of these markers if they are to play a diagnostic role in cancer. The Ph′, for example, while diagnostic for CML, is also found in other forms of leukaemia. It is possible that with the limitations of present banding techniques, the breakpoints giving rise to the Ph′ in CML are not identical to those forming the Ph′ in other forms of leukaemia. However, it is generally thought that the Ph′ is identical in all cancer and that induction of the Ph′ at different cell maturation stages would give rise to the different leukaemic diseases. There is an increased incidence of CML resulting from the atomic bombing in Japan, and the fact that ionizing radiation produced generally random chromosome damage suggests that the Ph′ is not the product of a site-specific carcinogen.

The role of chromosome analysis in cancer studies therefore remains somewhat equivocal. When pathological and clinical criteria are ambiguous chromosome studies may be of diagnostic value. Cells with altered chromosome complements provide strong evidence of a malignant condition, and their further evolution probably reflects the selection of cells with new malignant potential.

References

1. Boveri T: Zur Frage der Entstehung maligner tumoren. JENA Gustav Fischer 1914.
2. Winge O: Zytologische Untersuchungen über die Natur maligner Tumoren I. 'Crown Gall' der zucherrübe. Z Zellforsch 6:397–423, 1927.
3. Yoshida T: Studien über des 'Ascites-Sarcoma'. Proc Imp Acad Tokyo 20:611–620, 1944.
4. Levan A, Hauschka TS: Chromosome numbers of three mouse ascites tumours. Hereditas (Lund) 38:251–255, 1952.
5. Makino S: Further evidence favouring the concept of the stemline in ascites tumours of rats. Ann NY Acad Sci 63:818–830, 1956.
6. Spriggs AI, Boddington MM, Clarke CM: Carcinoma in-situ in the cervix uteri: some cytogenetic observations. Lancet i: 1383–1384, 1962.
7. Makino S, Ishihara T, Tonomura A: Cytological studies of tumours XXVII. The chromosomes of thirty human tumours. Z Krebforsch 63:184–208, 1959.
8. Hauschka TS: Correlation of chromosomal and physiological changes in tumours. J Cell Comp Physiol 52 (suppl. 1):197–233, 1958.
9. Hauschka TS, Levan A: Inverse relationship between chromosome ploidy and host specificity to sixteen transplantable tumours. Exp Cell Res 4:457–467, 1953.
10. Whang-Peng J, Knutson T, Ziegler J, Leventhal B: Cytogenetic studies in acute lymphocytic leukaemia: Special emphasis in long-term survival. Med Paediatr Oncol 2:333–351, 1976.
11. Sakurai M, Sandberg AA: Prognosis in acute myeloblastic leukaemia: chromosomal correlation. Blood 41:93–104, 1973.
12. Bloomfield CD, Peterson LC, Yunis JJ, Brunfield RD: The Philadelphia chromosome (Ph^1) in adults presenting with acute leukaemia: A comparison of Ph^1+ and Ph^1- patients. Br J Haematol 36:347–358, 1977.
13. Nowell PC, Hungerford DA: A minute chromosome in human chronic granulocytic leukaemia. Science 132:1497, 1960.
14. Rowley JD: A new consistent chromosomal abnormality in chronic myelogenous leukaemia identified by quinacrine fluorescence and Giemsa staining. Nature 243:290–293, 1973.
15. Sonta, SI, Sandberg AA: Chromosomes and causation of human cancer and leukaemia XXVIII. Value of detailed chromosome studies on large numbers of cells in CML. Am J Haematol 3:121–126, 1977.
16. Potter AM, Watmore AE, Cooke P, Lilleyman JS, Sokol RJ: Significance of non-standard Philadelphia chromosome in chronic granulocytic leukaemia. Br J Cancer 44:51–54, 1981.
17. Sakurai M, Sandberg AA: Chromosomes and causation of human cancer and leukaemia XVIII. The missing Y in acute myeloblastic leukaemia (AML) and Ph^1 positive myeloid leukaemia (CML). Cancer 38:762–769, 1976.
18. Finney R, McDonald GA, Baikie AG, Douglas AS: Chronic granulocytic leukaemia with Ph^1 negative cells and a ten year remission after busulphan hypoplasia. Br J Haematol 23:283–288, 1972.
19. Brandt L, Mitelman F, Panani A, Lenner HC: Extremely long duration of chronic myeloid leukaemia with Ph^1 negative and Ph^1 positive bone marrow cells. Scand J Haematol 16:321–325, 1976.
20. Fialkow PJ, Gartler SM, Yoshida A: Clonal origin of chronic myeloid leukaemia in man. Proc Natl Acad Sci USA 58:1468–1471, 1967.
21. Fitzgerald PH, Pickering AF, Eiby JR: Clonal origin of the Philadelphia chromosome and chronic myeloid leukaemia: Evidence from a sex chromosome mosaic. Br J Haematol 21:473–480, 1971.

22. Tough IM, Court Brown WM, Baikie AG, Buckton KE, Harnden DG, Jacobs PA, King MJ, McBride JA: Cytogenetic studies in chronic myeloid leukaemia and acute leukaemia associated with mongolism. Lancet i:411–417, 1961.
23. Lobb DS, Reeves BR, Lawler SD: Identification of isochromosome 17 in myeloid leukaemia. Lancet i:849–850, 1972.
24. Mitelman F, Levan G, Nilsson PG, Brandt L: Non-random karyotypic evolution in chronic myeloid leukaemia. Int J Cancer 18:24–30, 1976.
25. Prigogina EL, Fleischman EW, Volkova MA, Frenkel MA: Chromosome abnormalities and clinical and morphological manifestations of chronic myeloid leukaemia. Hum Genet 41:143–156, 1978.
26. Sonta SI, Sandberg AA: Chromosomes and the causation of human cancer and leukaemia XXIX. Further studies on the karyotypic progression of cancer in CML. Cancer 41:153–163, 1978.
27. Mitelman F, Levan G: Clustering of aberrations to specific chromosomes in human neoplasms III. Incidence and geographic distribution of chromosome aberrations in 856 cases. Hereditas 89:207–232, 1978.
28. Muller HJ: Artificial transmutation of the gene. Science 66:84–87, 1927.
29. Awa AA, Neriishi S, Honda T, Yoshida MC, Sofuni T, Matsui T: Chromosome-aberration frequency in cultured blood cells in relation to A-bomb survivors. Lancet ii:903–905, 1971.
30. Testa JR: Cytogenetic patterns in Polycythemia Vera. Cancer Genet Cytogenet I:207–215, 1980.
31. Honeycombe JR: The effects of busulphan on the chromosomes of normal human lymphocytes. Mutat Res 57:35–49, 1978.
32. Cohen MM, Shaw MW: Effects of mitomycin C on human chromosomes. J Cell Biol 23:386–395, 1964.
33. Morad M, Jonasson J, Lindsten J: Distribution of mitomycin C induced breaks on human chromosomes. Hereditas 74:273–282, 1973.
34. Rowley JD: Do human tumours show a chromosome pattern specific for each etiological agent? J Natl Cancer Inst 52:315–320, 1974.
35. Mitelman F, Levan G: The chromosomes of primary 7,12-dimethyl (α) anthracene induced rat sarcomas. Hereditas 71:325–334, 1972.

9. Tumour Immunology

R.C. REES and J.C.E. UNDERWOOD

1. Introduction

For many years it was thought that the apparently inexorable progression of malignant tumours could be halted or, at least, retarded only by surgical extirpation or other external influences. During this century, however, it has become clear that the growth of tumours may be subject to some internal controlling influences such as fluctuations in the endocrine milieu and immune responses. The role of immunological mechanisms in modulating tumour growth is the subject of this chapter. Immunity may operate against tumours as either an innate defence mechanism amenable to artificial therapeutic stimulation or as a factor working in concert with surgery, radiotherapy, and chemotherapy in a way that benefits the patient.

Despite the intensive study of tumour immunology during the last few decades, the knowledge gained currently has only very limited proven clinical relevance either to the diagnosis of cancer, its treatment, or the assessment of responses to therapy. However, the theoretical and experimental aspects invite detailed consideration because of the undeniable potential impact that tumour immunology could have on the clinical problem of cancer. Interest in tumour immunology has waxed and waned over the years, oscillating between unqualified pessimism and guarded optimism; the tenor of this review is cautiously optimistic about the future prospects for immunity and immunotherapy in the diagnosis and management of cancer in certain well-defined clinical situations.

2. Historical background

The first clue to the possible existence of some sort of naturally-occurring defence mechanism against cancer emerged from reports, admittedly anecdotal, of spontaneous regressions of proven human malignant neoplasms in the early years of the 20th century. These observations were the subject of the extensive review by Everson and Cole [1]. One must be cautious about uncritically accepting such cases as evidence favouring the existence of immunity to cancer until other possible causes for tumour regression (e.g.

Hancock, B. W. (ed.), Assessment of Tumour Response.
ISBN 90-247-2712-X.
Printed in The Netherlands.

infection, hormonal influences, occlusion of vascular supply) have been excluded.

Much animal experimentation was done between about 1900 and 1930 in an attempt to elucidate the nature of the immune response to tumours. The impetus for this work was largely derived from Ehrlich's pioneering observations that led to his 'athreptic' theory of tumour immunity. Most of these experiments involved tumour transplantation from one animal to another, the recipient animal often having been sensitised to the tumour by previous exposure; the tumour graft invariably regressed under such circumstances.

Little importance can now be credited to these observations. Woglom's highly critical review [2] was largely responsible for the abrupt curtailment of interest in experimental tumour immunology during the next decade. Prior to the introduction of inbred strains, experimental tumour immunology was conducted with outbred animals; any immune reaction or tumour rejection was probably provoked by ordinary histocompatability antigens and this early work thus provided no evidence for the existence of tumour-specific antigens.

The modern era of experimental tumour immunology dates from the observations of Gross [3], Foley [4] and Prehn and Main [5]. Using inbred mice that show identical histocompatability antigens they conclusively demonstrated the existence of novel antigens associated with transplantable tumours. Sensitisation to these tumour-specific antigens would protect the syngeneic mice against subsequent challenge with an otherwise tumourigenic dose of viable tumour cells.

Evidence for *human* tumour-specific antigens, and immune responses to them, is almost entirely circumstantial. This is understandable considering the insuperable ethical problems that would be otherwise involved. Among the earliest work is the observation that stromal infiltration by lymphoid cells confers a beneficial effect on patient survival; histological similarities with graft rejection reactions led to the conclusion that a similar immunological mechanism might be operating. This aspect is further discussed in the next section. In reviewing evidence for human tumour-associated antigens one must be cautious about 'antigens' discovered by raising antisera to human tumour tissue extracts in other species (e.g. carcinoembryonic antigen in colorectal carcinoma, etc.). These are substances found in tumours and detectable with heteroantisera; they may not be antigens in the strict operational sense of eliciting an immune response in the tumour-bearing host. Similarly, apparently tumour-specific antibodies must be rigorously assessed to exclude the possibility that they might merely be auto-antibodies to substances normally sequestered in healthy tissue (e.g. smooth muscle antibody, DNA antibodies). Subject to these caveats then, there does appear to be evidence for the existence of weakly immunogenic human tumour antigens and an immune reaction to them (see section 4.2).

For many years it has been fashionable to disregard apparently tumour-specific antibodies and to concentrate attention upon cell-mediated immunity. The reason for this is that, in experimental systems, the presence of immune serum antibody alone did not confer transplant immunity and was often adverse in its effect; the administration of such serum to tumour-bearing animals, or animals about to be challenged with tumour cells, often resulted in enhanced tumour growth [6, 7, 8]. More consistent protective effects were experienced with immune lymphoid cells. The discovery of cytotoxic or cytostatic effects of blood lymphoid cells on autologous tumour cells *in vitro,* reported by Hellstrom *et al.* [9] and others, spawned a vast amount of literature based on similar work. However, an exhaustive study by Takasugi *et al.* [10] showed that the cytotoxic effect of autologous lymphoid cells closely paralleled the effects of lymphoid cells from the blood of normal controls more often than had been formerly realised.

A thorough reappraisal of the *in vitro* studies in which blood lymphoid cells were added to tumour target cells has led to the view that there exists a subpopulation of cells in blood and lymphoid organs exhibiting innate cytolethal properties, to which neoplastic cells may be more susceptible than their normal counterparts. These are the so-called natural-killer (NK) cells [11] and are discussed in some detail in section 6.

3. Stromal reactions to cancer

Tumours are divisible into two cellular compartments: the neoplastic cell population itself and the connective tissue or stroma that supports it. The stroma comprises vascular channels conveying nutrition, fibrous tissue providing mechanical support, and variable proportions of lymphoreticular cells (i.e. for the purposes of this discussion – lymphocytes, macrophages, polymorphonuclear leukocytes, and mast cells) (Fig. 1).

Although the presence of lymphoreticular cells in the stroma of tumours was recognised by Virchow, he attributed them to pre-existing inflammation at sites of cancer development. In the 1920s McCarty and his colleagues noted that patients with gastric and mammary cancer whose tumours harboured dense lymphoid infiltrates survived longer than those patients whose tumours were virtually devoid of infiltration. This observation has been repeated on many occasions for these and other tumours [12]. Some tumours that characteristically bear dense lymphoreticular infiltrates, such as medullary carcinoma of the breast and seminoma of the testis, have a notably good prognosis. However, this prognostic advantage is not absolutely clear-cut and an adverse effect has occasionally been recorded.

The histological appearances of densely infiltrated tumours bear a resemblance at the light-microscopic level to rejecting experimental tumours and

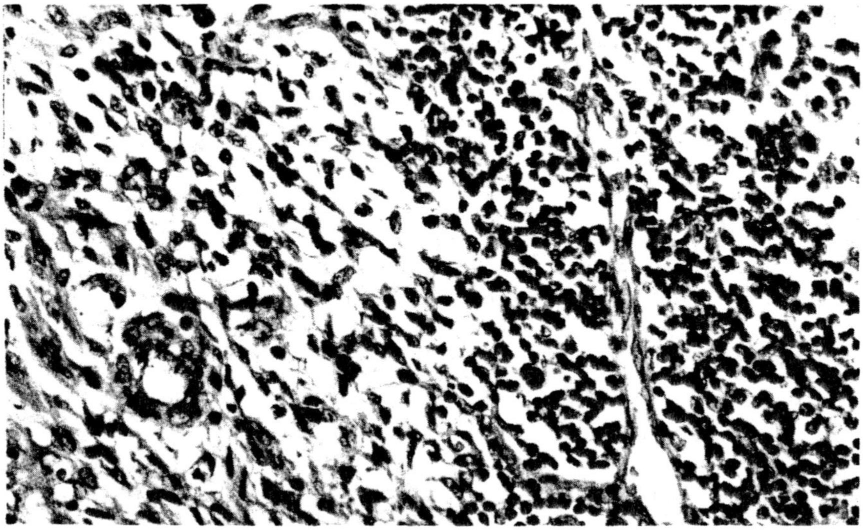

Figure 1. Dense perivascular lymphocytic infiltrate in a myxoid liposarcoma. This appearance may be seen within and in the immediate vicinity of many human tumours and in some instances positively correlates with prognosis (Haematoxylin and Eosin × 240).

organ grafts. This has led to speculation that perhaps the infiltrates might signal host immunity and possibly be actually engaged in destruction of tumour cells. However, detailed ultrastructural studies [13] have failed to provide any direct morphological evidence of cytotoxic interactions between neoplastic cells and the lymphoreticular cells permeating the stroma, though the two cell populations are often in close apposition. Similarly, lymphoid cells extracted from tumours are apparently devoid of reactivity against cultured autologous tumour cells [14].

These findings contrast with observations in Hodgkin's lymphoma in which the relative proportion of lymphocytes to the putative neoplastic cells (Reed-Sternberg cells, abnormal reticulum cells) also correlates with prognosis. In this condition ultrastructural studies provide morphological evidence of possible toxic interactions between lymphocytes and other cells [15].

Technical problems limit the amount of useful information that can be gleaned from direct study of tumour tissue. The precise nature of the immune response to human and experimental tumours is the subject of continuing observations of the anti-tumour effects of lymphoid cells from the blood and lymphoid organs.

4. Tumour antigens

The antigenic changes accompanying neoplasia are of considerable importance in relation to both immunotherapy and immunodiagnosis. Many of the 'new' products present on or secreted from cancer cells are, however, incapable of eliciting an immune response in the autologous syngeneic host and although of potential importance in diagnosis and monitoring disease progression they are of little value in controlling tumour growth *in vivo* and the functional significance of many of these tumour products is not known. Many experimental tumours express a 'tumour rejection antigen(s)'. Before discussing the evidence for the presence of tumour antigens on human cancer cells, the nature and biological importance of tumour associated transplantation antigens (TATA) of experimental tumours will be considered; in the past results from experimental studies have provided valuable guidelines in a search for human TATA.

4.1. Tumour antigens associated with experimental tumours

In essence, the presence of a tumour associated transplantation antigen (TATA) can only be demonstrated *in vivo,* where prior immunisation against a specific tumour elicits immunity to tumour challenge with live tumour-producing doses of homologous cells. Detection of tumour associated antigenic determinants using *in vitro* methods, fails to establish these as rejection antigens. Table 1 summarises the TATA associated with experimental neoplasia. To determine the presence of rejection antigens, tests are performed in inbred animal strains where individual tumours can be maintained *in vivo* by serial passage. Immunisation by inoculation of attenuated tumour cell or antigen preparations, or by tumour graft resection (Table 2),

Table 1. Transplantation rejection antigens associated with experimental tumours

Tumours	Antigen(s)	Specificity	Reference
Chemically-induced rodent tumours	TATA	Usually individually tumour specific	27
DNA-virus-induced rodent tumours	TATA	Virus specific	27
Murine leukaemias	TL	–	126
Oncornavirus-induced avian and feline tumours	TSA	–	127, 128
Murine leukaemia virus-induced (Friend Moloney and Rauscher viruses)	TATA	–	129
Spontaneously arising tumours	TATA	Individually specific. Many tumours are non-specific	21, 22

Table 2. Immunisation procedures used to elicit a transplantation rejection response

Immunisation	Comments
Attenuated (X-irradiated) tumour cells/tissue	Used in most tumour systems.
Tumour graft resection	With non-metastasising tumours.
Solubilised TATA (cell-free tumour homogenates)	Only with certain DNA-virus-induced and chemically-induced tumours.
Virus-immunisation	By immunisation of adult animals with live oncogenic DNA viruses (abortive transformation).

is carried out before tumour cell challenge; the failure of tumours to appear in immunised, as compared with control (non-immunised), animals is taken to indicate the presence of a TATA(s).

The specificity of TATA in carcinogen-induced tumours has been studied in some detail. In the main these neoplasms express an individually specific TATA, and the view is held that these represent depressed or mutated gene products. In contrast, DNA-virus induced tumours express a TATA common to all tumours induced with the same virus. Exceptions occur where some chemically-induced tumours have been found to express a cross-reacting rejection antigen, in addition to an individually-specific component [16, 17, 18]. The nature of the cross-reacting determinants has not been established, but they may represent the re-expression in neoplasia of fetal antigens which are recognised by the host as non-self [19, 20].

Many rodent sarcomas and carcinomas induced with polycyclic hydrocarbons, are known to possess a TATA capable of evoking a strong tumour rejection response; high immunogenicity is associated with tumours induced with high doses of carcinogen. Some chemically-induced neoplasms lack a detectable TATA(s) altogether and spontaneously arising animal tumours are, in the main, weakly or non-immunogenic [21–24]. Analogies have been drawn, although not proven, between human tumours and spontaneously arising animal tumours [25, 26].

The *in vivo* assays used to demonstrate tumour rejection do not allow for quantitation of the TATA, and attempts to establish a reliable *in vitro* assay for tumour antigens have met with only mild success. Most assays such as macrophage migration inhibition and indirect immunofluorescence rely heavily on the use of solubilised tumour antigen. In some systems solubilised tumour antigen has been found to elicit an *in vivo* tumour rejection response [6, 27]. Detergent solubilised associated TATA of a BALB/c mouse Mc-induced sarcoma has been shown to elicit specific transplantation immunity to challenge with live Meth A tumour cells [27, 28]. The transplantation activity of 3M KCl extracts of other chemically-induced murine sarcomas has also been achieved, but such preparations appear effective only within a narrow dose range [29–31].

Not all tumour antigens associated with rodent tumours elicit transplant immunity when presented to the host in a soluble or subcellular form. Extensive studies using rat hepatoma and sarcoma models have given contrasting results [7, 8, 32]. In these studies isolated tumour cell plasma membranes, or membrane antigen(s) solubilised by papain and ionic or non-ionic detergents, while retaining the capacity to specifically neutralise antitumour antibody in membrane immunofluorescence, complement fixation or isotopic anti-globulin assays, failed to induce immunity to homologous tumour cell challenge. With these tumours transplantation resistance was only shown for animals immunised with intact X-irradiated tumour cell vaccines, although serum antibody could be demonstrated in rats immunised with sub-cellular tumour cell components. The mode of presentation, and processing of antigen *in vivo* may therefore be critical in the successful initiation of transplant immunity (see section 5).

With tumours of RNA viral aetiology the expression of tumour-related cell surface antigens is more complex than with other experimental tumours. Besides expressing a TATA, these tumours have a wide ranging complex of virus associated products, for example gp 70, p30 and p15 viral antigens are expressed in transformed cells. Many of the viral structural antigens are incorporated into the glycocalyx of the cell membrane, and may act as recognition sites, triggering host defence mechanisms to produce tumour rejection. Kurth *et al.* [33] have recently reviewed antigen expression in tumours induced by RNA viruses, and these will not be discussed further here.

4.2. Tumour antigens associated with human tumours

Although tumour antigen(s) expression on experimental tumours has been firmly established, the presence of similar components of tumour related specificity has not been demonstrated on human tumours. Neoantigen expression in human neoplasia has relied heavily on the use of *in vitro* assays, such as those listed in Table 3. Of the experimental tests employed to demonstrate host reactivity to tumour antigens, *in vitro* cytotoxicity assays have been widely used.

Claims of organ related tumour antigens stemmed from work pioneered by the Hellstroms, initially using the colony inhibition assay [34] and subsequently the 48–72 h micro-cytotoxicity test [35]. The results of these studies were originally interpreted as demonstrating the expression, at the cell surface of human cancer cells, of individually specific and organ specific tumour antigens, to which the host mounted a predominantly cell-mediated

Table 3. Assays for detecting tumour immune responses

Assays for demonstrating host sensitisation

i Skin testing (*in vivo*) using soluble 'tumour antigen'.
ii Leukocyte/Macrophage Migration Inhibition using tumour cells, isolated membrane or solublised 'tumour antigen'.
iii Leukocyte Adherence Inhibition.
iv Blastogenic responses of peripheral blood T-lymphocytes to autologous mitomycin-C treated tumour cells.

Assays demonstrating host cytotoxic responses

i Short–Medium term (4–18 h) isotope release tests against autologous tumour targets.

immune response. With our further understanding of the ways in which lymphoid cells and their products influence tumour cells in culture, less reliance was placed on the initial interpretation of results obtained using these assays; not least was the finding that peripheral blood lymphocytes displayed natural antitumour cytotoxicity [11]. It is pertinent that studies in rodents have shown that normal host lymphoid cells in culture generate factors capable of promoting and retarding the growth of tumour cells in culture [36].

In spite of inherent difficulties associated with this, and other laboratory tests designed to show host reactivity to tumour associated antigens, extensive studies have been undertaken to investigate this important question, using a variety of immunological techniques [37–42]. At best, the results from these studies show that some, but not all, patients possess reactivity to an autologous and possibly allogeneic tumour antigen(s).

Lymphocytes from patients with tumours of differing histology, have been shown to undergo blastogenesis in co-culture with autologous tumour cells, and to develop autologous cytotoxicity against tumour targets [42–45], thus suggesting that host lymphocytes are sensitised to autologous tumour cell antigens. It is pertinent to note that the presence of sensitising tumour antigens may not necessarily mean the presence of an antigen capable of evoking a tumour rejection response, and acting as a target determinant for host mediated tumour rejection.

In vivo skin testing has been used in attempts to show the presence of human tumour specific antigens [46, 47], although studies of this nature are hampered by ethical considerations. Another approach which has been adopted to establish the existence of human tumour antigens has been to prepare xenogeneic antiserum against human tumours, and remove antibody reactivity to normal cell components by extensive absorption/neutralisation with normal host cells. These studies have yielded results which have been interpreted as indicating the presence of human tumour antigens;

in some instances these may represent normal differentiation antigens not normally detectable in normal adult tissue [48]. Difficulties are however encountered with this approach, and such antisera may possess reactivity directed against normal cell components present in low concentrations on many cells. A second approach has been to use sera from cancer patients to determine the presence of antibodies reactive towards antigens of established *in vitro* human tumour cell lines, but this is plagued with the difficulty of determining the contribution of alloantibodies to the observed reactions, and results obtained using this methodology must be viewed with some caution.

Using tests based on the autologous serological typing of cultured target cells, recent studies by Shiku *et al.* [49] have inferred the presence of three distinct classes of antigen associated with human malignant melanomas, astrocytomas and renal carcinomas. The possible existence in human tumours of individually specific, shared tumour-specific, and widely distributed cell-surface tumour-associated components was suggested from the results. However, biochemical characterisation is required to evaluate the relationship of these antigens to other cell components, particularly those associated with the major histocompatibility complex. At this point in time, the critical issue of whether human tumours possess antigens capable of evoking relevant host immunity, and subsequently acting as targets for tumour cell destruction, has not been resolved. The preparation of monoclonal antibodies against tumour antigens may prove helpful in defining more precisely the inherent nature of human tumour antigens. Although this approach may prove of value in establishing the presence of specific or common tumour cell components, it will fall short of establishing their *in vivo* significance.

5. Tumour specific immune responses

The initiation of specific transplant immunity is dependent on the tumour expressing antigens capable of promoting the relevant immune response in the autologous/syngeneic host. Much of our current knowledge of transplantation resistance has come from animal studies, where it has proved possible to observe tumour directed immune responses in syngeneic inbred strains of mice and rats. In humans, little information is available defining either the presence of a tumour rejection antigen(s) or the nature of the rejection response, and our discussion will be confined mainly to observations in experimental tumour systems.

Although several tumour-related antigens may be expressed at the tumour cell surface few, if any, will be capable of initiating tumour immunity; the ultimate test for this is the rejection of a tumour-producing inoculum of tumour cells. Table 2 lists the most commonly used methods for the induction of transplantation resistance, and on the basis of the results from these assays, tumours can be classified as strong, weak or non-immunogenic. Tumours induced by administration of chemical carcinogens or oncogenic DNA-viruses, usually evoke a relatively strong tumour immune response, and it is interesting to speculate whether tumours of weaker immunogenicity possibly induce adverse host responses, or secrete products which subvert either the induction or reactive phase of the immunity. The effectiveness of the immune response in tumour rejection may therefore be dependent on the balance between immunological activation and suppression.

In discussing the *in vivo* relevance of tumour immunity, antigenic heterogeneity within the primary tumour and its metastatic deposits is of prime importance. Immunogenic differences have been observed between the primary tumour and distal metastases [50, 51, 52]. Concomitant immunity might therefore lead to the development of tumours which metastasise, showing either a loss or change in TATA's [53]. Indeed recent studies suggest that the host milieu may augment the generation of tumour heterogeneity [54]. Antigenic differences between primary and secondary tumours have also been demonstrated *in vitro* using specifically activated cytotoxic T-lymphocytes [55, 56], and strengthens the view that cells of different immunogenicity co-exist within the primary tumour.

Clearly, established lines of thought favour the concept that in solid tumours cell-mediated rather than the humoral limb of the host response is the prime mechanism of tumour rejection, although antitumour antibody may play an important role in immunity towards leukaemic cells [57]. Whether human tumours possess TATA's capable of evoking specific host responses is critical to the application of specific immunotherapy in the control of human malignant disease and central to this issue is the possible heterogeneity or absence of rejection antigens particularly in metastatic deposits. The major effector mechanisms operative against tumours are summarised in Fig. 2.

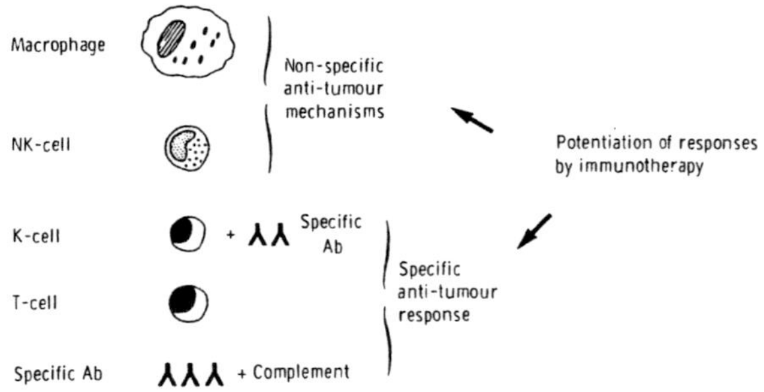

Figure 2. Host mediated anti-tumour responses.

6. Natural cell-mediated reactivity against tumours

The existence of a particular subpopulation of lymphoid cells possessing innate reactivity (cytotoxicity) towards cancer cells, represents one of the most exciting discoveries of the last decade. The principal effector cell population has been termed the natural killer (NK) cell [11] and much work has focused on defining the specificity of reactivity, characterisation of the effector cell population, immunoregulation/modulation of killing, and the relationship of this mechanism to tumour growth inhibition and immune surveillance *in vivo.*

6.1. *Historical*

Early attempts to establish the existence of tumour specific antigens on human tumours were hampered by the techniques available. Much criticism has since been made of the colony inhibition [34] and microcytotoxicity tests [35], and it became apparent that these long-term cytotoxicity assays had many shortcomings, the most important being the effect of normal (non-sensitised) lymphoid cells and their products in inhibiting or stimulating tumour growth [36]. The interpretation of the results from these tests was somewhat dependent on the level of target cell growth enhancement/inhibition in the presence of lymphoid cells from normal individuals. Subsequently, and with the development of the short term (4–6 h) ^{51}Chromium-release assay [58], reports on the antitumour reactivity of normal individuals began to emerge [59, 60, 61]. At this time also, animal studies showed the existence of NK cells to be a general phenomenon [62, 63, 64] affirming the wider significance of natural killing. Indeed the true significance of NK cells and their role as antiviral and homeostatic control mechanisms has only recently been considered [65, 66].

6.2. *Characterisation of NK and related cytotoxic effector cells*

NK cells have been extensively studied in mice, rats and humans; definition of their cell lineage has relied on analysis of their physical and biological properties relative to other, well-characterised, lymphoid sub-populations. Most of these studies have been carried out using human and animal leukaemia cells as targets, although NK reactivity towards solid tumour targets has been demonstrated [67]. *In vivo* cultured leukaemia cells are particularly susceptible to NK-cell killing, and most studies have utilised effector cells isolated from the peripheral blood or spleen, where relatively high levels of NK reactivity are to be found.

In addition, cytotoxicity has been shown in cells isolated from the peritoneum and to a lesser extent the lymph nodes, reactivity being absent in the thymus and bone marrow [11].

The suggestion that NK cells may be of T-cell lineage comes from studies showing NK effectors to express T-cell surface markers. Some human NK cells form low affinity E-rosettes with sheep erythrocytes [68], although a subpopulation of cytotoxic cells is non-E rosetting (E^-).

It is now generally agreed that human and rodent NK cells express receptor sites for the Fc portion of immunoglobulin (FcR^+), a feature commonly associated with K cells and phagocytic macrophages and monocytes. NK cells can be further distinguished from mature T-cells by the fact that T-cell cytotoxicity requires identity with its target in antigens expressed by the major histocompatibility complex (MHC-restriction) in addition to the appropriate specific sensitisation to the target antigen. The cytotoxicity mediated by NK cells is not MHC-restricted, and NK-sensitive allogeneic (and in some instances xenogeneic) target cells show high susceptibility to killing. Also, the observation that congenitally athymic mice and rats, which are devoid of mature T-lymphocytes, possess high levels of NK cells, serves to distinguish NK cells from mature circulating T-lymphocytes.

Further evidence indicates that NK cells are of separate lineage to B-lymphocytes, by virtue of the fact that NK cells fail to show the presence of surface membrane immunoglobulin, Ia antigens, or C3 receptors, which are normally associated with B-lymphocytes [69]. NK cells also lack the properties of mature macrophages and monocytes, since they are glass and plastic non-adherent, and are eluted from nylon wool columns [11].

6.3. Immunomodulation of NK activity

It has recently become clear that the cytolytic activity of cells can be augmented above basal levels by several agents including viruses, synthetic polynucleotides, bacterial products, tumour cells, interferon and interferon inducers [70–74]. Considerable attention has been given to the role of interferon (IF) in potentiating NK activity, and it is generally agreed that IF is one of the major mediators of NK augmentation. The agents listed above and shown to modulate NK activity are themselves capable of inducing type I (lymphoblastoid or α IF) and in some cases type II (fibroblast or β IF) following *in vitro* incubation with lymphoid cells or administration *in vivo*. For example, Bacillus Calmette Guérin (BCG) and Corynebacterium parvum (*C. parvum*) cause significant boosting of NK cell activity, initiating the production of type I IF in some cases from accessory macrophage cells.

Human α and β IF augments spontaneous cytotoxicity of human NK cells isolated from peripheral blood in a dose-dependent manner, and although

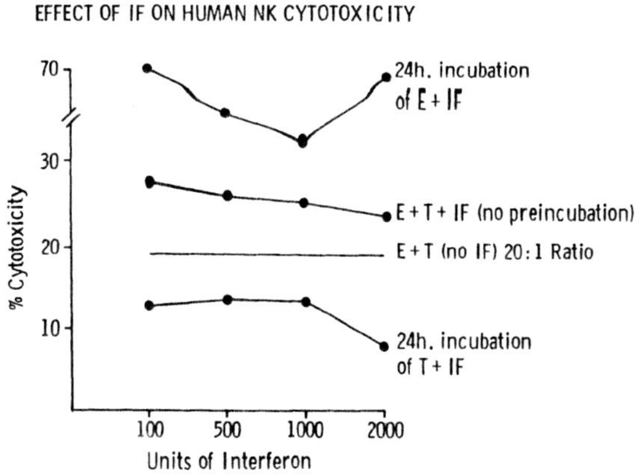

Figure 3. Influence of α interferon on cytotoxicity mediated by human NK cells, and target resistance to NK cytolysis. Target cells = K562, Effector cells = Human Nylon wool non-adherent PBL. Results from a four hour ^{51}Cr-release assay.
Pretreatment of effector cells with α IF causes significant enhancement of NK cytotoxicity, whilst pretreatment of K562 target cells induces a degree of resistance to NK cell killing which may be due to alterations in the efficiency of target cell repair mechanisms.

only a short exposure to IF is necessary to initiate boosting of cytotoxicity, increased reactivity does not become apparent following increased (1–2 h) pre-treatment of effectors (Fig. 3). Recent studies have shown that IF mediates its effect on NK cells in two distinct ways (Timonen, Ortaldo and Herberman, unpublished results). First, IF causes recruitment of precursor NK cells to mature cytotoxic effectors, increasing the proportion of NK effector cells binding to targets and causing target cell lysis. Secondly, IF has also been shown to increase the kinetics of cytolysis of individual NK cells. One can speculate that endogenous production of IF *in vivo* is important in the development and maintenance of spontaneous levels of NK reactivity, although evidence for this is at present lacking. It is clear from studies to date that IF is capable of regulating the level of NK cell antitumour reactivity [75].

6.4. *In vivo relevance of NK cells*

Many of our ideas as to the *in vivo* role of NK cells come from observations in experimental animal systems; the findings have in general supported the idea that NK effector cells play a central role in immune surveillance against cancer and the rapid elimination of tumour cells *in vivo.* Recent observations fail to encourage belief in the concept that immune surveillance is mediated by a thymus-dependent (T-lymphocyte) host response to tumour associated antigens [76]. In particular, congenitally athymic (Nu^+/Nu^+) nude mice have been shown to develop spontaneous tumours at the same rate as their euthymic, immunologically intact, litter-mates [77]. Further evidence suggesting that host resistance to neoplasia is dependent on a functionally intact NK system is inferred from studies in mice using IF Chimeras reconstituted with bone marrow cells derived from mice with high or low NK reactivity, where NK sensitive, but not insensitive, T-lymphomas were subject to growth suppression when injected *in vivo* [78]. Other studies have also correlated high NK reactivity with tumour resistance [79, 80].

The influence of tumour growth on NK cell reactivity should also be considered. In mice bearing primary virus-induced or transplanted tumours, systemic NK activity has been shown to be decreased [81, 82, 83] and in some human studies results have shown cancer patients to have a reduced level of NK activity [84, 85, 86], although this has not proved to be the case with all types of cancers [87]. Whether the observed reduction in NK cell activity is due to a reduction in the number of effector cells or a reduced cytolytic capability of individual NK cells is not known. The demonstration of systemic NK activity may not reflect immunological events at the tumour site, and several groups of researchers have tried, without success, to isolate and identify host cells mediating spontaneous antitumour cytotoxicity from within the tumour [88, 89, 90]. If one accepts that the isolation procedures used are efficient in recovering functionally active NK cells, then it may be concluded that either NK effector cells fail to infiltrate human tumours, or they become inactivated as a result of immunosuppression by tumour products or as a consequence of interaction with target cells. An important finding with regard to this last supposition has been the demonstration that NK cell-tumour-cell interaction can not only lead to the death of the target cell, but also a decrease in the cytolytic capacity of re-isolated effector cells. Effective neutralisation of cytotoxic host cells therefore represents an important escape mechanism for the tumour [91]. It has also been suggested that interferon activated NK cells are capable of retaining their cytotoxic capability following binding and release from target cells [91], and this finding may be important with regard to the use of interferon or interferon inducers in cancer therapy.

6.5. Natural cytotoxic (NC) cells

Stutman *et al.* [92] have reported a cytotoxic murine lymphocyte population reactive towards a chemically-induced fibrosarcoma of BALB/c origin [93, 94], and distinguished this cell type from NK cells, inferring heterogeneity within the 'natural defence' system. Whereas NK cells manifest their cytotoxicity within 4–6 h of co-culture with susceptible target cells, NC reactivity is only apparent following an 18 h culture period with target cells derived from solid tumours. It has also been shown that NC, unlike

NK cells are present at birth and persist into old age, and are relatively resistant to treatments which depress spontaneous NK cytotoxicity, e.g. *in vivo* administration of cyclophosphamide, carrageenan and silica. The demonstration of NC cell reactivity is restricted to the observations with murine fibrosarcomas, and progress in this field awaits confirmation of this finding in other tumour systems.

6.6. Natural macrophage cytotoxicity

The spontaneous antitumour cytotoxicity mediated by monocytes and macrophages may also act as an immune surveillance system. Attention has focussed on the tumouricidal capacity of spontaneous and 'activated' cells of the monocyte-macrophage series. Tumour cell lysis *in vitro* by phagocytic cells can be demonstrated using a 24–48 h cytotoxicity assay, and is subject to interferon-dependent and independent immunopotentiation by biological stimulants. Under suitable test conditions, both direct cytolysis and cytostasis can be shown, and although the precise mechanism of cell destruction remains obscure, toxicity is thought to involve cell–cell contact and the production of cytotoxic oxidants, e.g. H_2O_2 and O_2, and/or proteases; cytostasis, however, may involve the production of prostaglandins which regulate cell growth. In addition, macrophages may also release soluble cytolytic products, causing tumour cell lysis without the necessity for conjugation with target cells [97, 98].

Macrophages may regulate several other immune-functions and are thought to play a central role in the development and maintenance of NK cell activity. Alternatively macrophages can suppress lymphoproliferation, lymphokine production, the generation of cytotoxic T-cells, and suppress NK activity, possibly through the release of prostaglandins.

7. Immune modulation and tumour growth

Despite the persuasive evidence that the body is capable of mounting an immune response to tumours, cancer still remains a major clinical problem; it seems that the tumour evades destruction despite the possibility that many are recognised as an immunogenic tissue. This interplay between tumour and host at an immunological level merits further consideration in two ways: first, the occurrence and behaviour of tumours in immunosuppressed hosts; second, the subversion of antitumour immune reactivity in tumour-bearing hosts.

7.1. Tumours in immunosuppressed hosts

The extensive use of immunosuppressive agents in the management of patients with renal and other transplants led to the recognition that such patients have an unexpectedly higher incidence of neoplasms than comparable controls. It is tempting to conclude that this might be due to the abrogation of an immunosurveillance system against neoplasia. However, two pieces of evidence suggest that this general conclusion cannot be drawn.

The incidence of tumours in carcinogen-treated animals shows no constant correlation with their level of innate immunity. A wide variety of suppressive agents or the use of athymic ('nude') mice have failed to show any permissive effect of immune impairment on tumour development. Indeed, many of these experimental models of immune impairment are more resistant to carcinogenic agents than are their counterparts with normal immunity [99]. These findings are contrary to the precepts of a general immunosurveillance theory.

Statistical analysis of the data from patients who have developed neoplasms during treatment with immunosuppressives has shown that only two tumour types are present in excess: these are lymphomas and cutaneous squamous cell carcinomas [100]. This raises the possibility that certain immunosuppressive agents may have a direct oncogenic effect on lymphoid tissue and squamous epithelium.

7.2. Subversion of antitumour immunity

Although the immunosurveillance theory is conceptually attractive, there is no evidence that in fact specific immune responses play any part in controlling oncogenesis. This does not, though, mean that immunity is incapable of resisting the growth of fully established immunogenic tumours. The

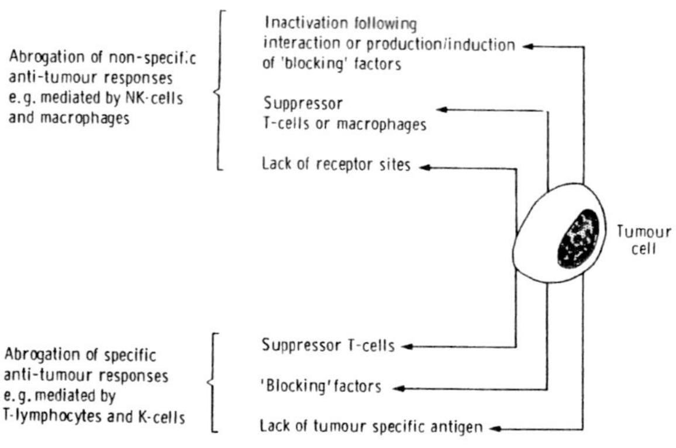

Figure 4. Escape mechanisms.

possible existence of cytotoxic lymphoid cells in the blood of cancer patients, for example, suggests evidence for a potentially defensive reaction against the tumour, but there is little evidence that this is effective *in vivo*. It is thus possible that antitumour immunoreactivity may be subverted *in vivo* through either specific or nonspecific mechanisms which are potentiated as a result of tumour development (Fig. 4).

Various humoral agents have been proposed to explain the escape from specific antitumour immunity; these include antitumour antibody (masking antigenic sites on the tumour cell surface), excess tumour antigen (masking specific immunoglobulin associated with the surface of immune cells), and antigen–antibody complexes [101]. Evidence for such blocking factors came from early studies in which lymphocytes in the blood of cancer patients were found to be cytotoxic towards cultured autologous tumour cells. The addition of autologous serum to these *in vitro* systems often specifically abrogated the cytotoxic interactions. These phenomena might explain the specific failure of antitumour immune reactivity, but it would not explain the generalised anergic state of many cancer patients demonstrable either by skin testing with a wide range of recall antigens or by seeking sensitisation to novel allergens such as dinitrochlorobenzene (DNCB). To explain this we must invoke some nonspecific subversive system.

Many substances have now been shown to be capable of suppressing lymphocyte function *in vitro* in a nonspecific fashion. These include α-fetoprotein, human chorionic gonadotrophin, fibrin degradation products, pregnancy-associated macroglobulin, prostaglandins, etc. [102]. In some cancer patients the concentration of these factors exhibiting immunomodulatory effects correlates with the anergic state as determined by delayed hypersensitivity skin testing [102]. It is conceivable that some other factors, as yet poorly characterised, may be derived from macrophages actually infiltrating the tumour tissue.

The role to T-suppressor cells is currently under investigation [99]. This subclass of T-lymphocytes serves to modulate lymphocyte reactivity towards specific antigens and could explain the specific suppression of antitumour immunity.

8. Immunodiagnosis of cancer

A wide variety of immunological methods have been used in the diagnosis and further assessment of cancer patients [103]. We shall not, however, consider further in this chapter tumour-associated substances (e.g. carcinoembryonic antigen, ferritin, hormones) that were originally detected or are now measured by immunological methods such as radio-immunoassay; these tumour markers are the subject of Chapter 6.

The principle underlying the diagnostic methods to be discussed here is that detectable sensitisation of peripheral blood lymphoid cells to tumour-associated antigens may indicate the presence of tumour in an individual patient. A prerequisite is the availability of a reasonably well-characterised panel of tumour antigen and normal tissue antigen preparations that can be used in the various tests; these are cell or tissue extracts used in either a crude or, preferably, purified state. These diagnostic tests have been conducted *in vivo* or *in vitro* (Table 2).

In vivo testing involves seeking cutaneous delayed hypersensitivity reactions to tissue extracts. If the growth of tumours was constantly associated with immune recognition of their presence it should be possible to elicit visible skin reactions to injections of appropriate antigenic material [104]. In all these tests it is desirable to use antigens that are common to all tumours of a certain histogenetic type rather than antigens that are rarely shared by different tumours of the same type.

A variety of *in vitro* tests have been proposed. They frequently have a common history; the laboratory responsible for discovering the test usually finds a high degree of accuracy (few false negatives or false positives) but other laboratories often fail to reproduce these findings [105]. Some of the tests are exquisitely sensitive to apparently trivial perturbations in ambient conditions in the laboratory and rigourous attention to the preparation of glassware, buffers, etc. is usually essential. However, these tests hold tremendous promise for the diagnosis of early cancer.

8.1. Lymphocyte transformation

If sensitised lymphocytes are exposed to specific antigen they undergo functional and morphological changes; DNA synthesis and mitotic activity occurs, B-lymphocytes differentiate into immunoglobulin-secreting cells and T-lymphocytes generate lymphokines. The mitogenic effect of antigens on sensitised lymphocytes can be measured by assessing the incorporation of ^{3}H-thymidine into DNA. Thus if a patient harbours an immunogenic tumour, circulating lymphocytes will transform on exposure to the appropriate tumour antigen.

8.2. Macrophage migration inhibition

Transformed T-lymphocytes secrete a variety of humoral factors (lymphokines), one of which – macrophage inhibitory factor (MIF) – retards the innate tendency of macrophages to migrate across the surface of a culture vessel and is probably important in mediating the accumulation of macrophages in inflamed tissue. In the MIF assay, peripheral blood buffy coat is packed into an open tube which is then placed on a culture surface and covered with medium; the macrophages in the buffy coat migrate to form a fan-shaped zone around the end of the tube. If the buffy-coat cells come from a patient sensitised to an immunogenic tumour the zone of migration will be smaller when tumour extract is present in the culture medium.

8.3. Macrophage electrophoretic mobility

This controversial test relies upon the ability of transformed T-lymphocytes to secrete a factor that modifies the unidirectional movement of monocytes and macrophages in an electrical field. The appropriate lymphokine reduces the mobility of the macrophages. This MEM test was originally used to test for sensitisation to an encephalitogenic factor in patients with demyelinating diseases, but it was subsequently claimed to be a sensitive and accurate diagnostic test for the presence of cancer [106]. Other workers have been unable to reproduce the original claims for this method despite strict adherence to the experimental protocols and conditions [105].

8.4. Leucocyte adherence inhibition

Halliday and his colleagues [107] discovered that the natural tendency of lymphoid cells to lightly adhere to certain surfaces, notably glass, was inhibited when such cells were suspended in a medium containing an antigen to which they were sensitised. Like some of the other tests already considered in this section the method is remarkably fickle and not all laboratories are able to achieve the accuracy and sensitivity attributed to it. The LAI test has nevertheless generated much interest because it is relatively rapid and the experimental manipulations and cell-counting procedures would lend themselves to automation.

9. Prospects for immunotherapy

A logical extension of research into tumour immunology, and indeed the motivation for such research, is the development of immunological methods for the treatment of cancer. To date, however, immunotherapy of human cancer has not proved to be universally or consistently successful though encouraging results have been obtained [108]. Experimental schedules can be devised in animal models in which immunisation will protect against an otherwise tumourigenic inoculum; regression of an established tumour is less easy to achieve. As with so much in tumour immunology, extrapolation from animal models to the human cancer problem is rarely simple. For those seeking more information on the history of immunotherapy the review by Currie [109] is recommended.

Even in tumours which have been shown to be amenable to immunotherapy it does have a restricted clinical role. Immunotherapy is ineffective against a large tumour burden such as that which is present in the patient with clinically evident cancer. It is most effective when the bulk of the tumor has been dealt with by surgery, radiotherapy or chemotherapy and only traces of disease like clinically occult metastases remain to be eradicated. The advantages of immunotherapy are that, first, unlike surgery or radiotherapy it has the potential when systemically administered to gain access to widely disseminated disease and, secondly, unlike most conventional chemotherapy, its efficacy is largely independent of cell-cycle kinetics.

It is convenient to consider nonspecific and specific immunotherapy separately.

9.1. Nonspecific immunotherapy

In the 1920s Coley noted that tumours sometimes regressed when they became infected, or if infection was present in the vicinity. More recently it has been shown that postoperative empyema after thoracotomy and resection for lung cancer is associated with improved survival [110]. The beneficial therapeutic effect appears to be mediated by nonspecific mechanisms; macrophages and NK cells are the probable effector cells.

The most widely used agents for nonspecific immunotherapy are BCG, *Corynebacterium parvum,* levamisole, and more recently, interferons. The idea of using bacteria originates from Coley's toxin, a tumour vaccine composed of a cocktail of killed bacteria.

BCG was first employed in the treatment of acute leukaemia by Mathé and his colleagues [111]. However, the encouraging results claimed by this early study have not been matched by the results from other trials and the undoubted therapeutic benefit stemming from advances in chemotherapy has now overtaken the questionable additional advantages of adjuvant immunotherapy for leukaemia.

One of the most effective applications of BCG immunotherapy has been in lung cancer. Intrapleural BCG (one dose of 10^7 organisms given postoperatively after tumour resection) resulted in a 93% disease free rate at 2 years compared with 67% disease free rate in randomised cases treated by resection alone [112].

BCG may also be given intralesionally in tumours that are accessible, skin tumours for example. Up to 90% of skin metastases from malignant melanoma will regress after intralesional injection of BCG; concomitant regression of uninjected lesions is also occasionally seen [113].

Mild fever and malaise with ulceration of the injection site are not unexpected side-effects of BCG administration. BCG can, however, be hazardous if systemic infection or anaphylaxis occurs [114]. Also there is some evidence that low-dose BCG therapy may actually accelerate tumour growth in some patients with malignant melanoma and many of the early studies are questionable because of the use of historical or non-randomised controls [115]. Certainly BCG merits further consideration for use as a nonspecific immunotherapeutic agent but caution must be exercised in the interpretation of published data from the clinical trials so far conducted.

Likewise the results of clinical trials of *Corynebacterium parvum,* administered by intravenous or subcutaneous injection, have shown only marginal or doubtful benefit when used as an adjuvant in patients with disseminated malignant melanoma, breast carcinoma and ovarian carcinoma [108]. Levamisole, an antihelminthic agent, has been less intensively studied in clinical trials, but here too the results are now of borderline significance [115] despite early optimism [116].

There has been, of late, considerable interest in interferon as an anticancer drug; the effect of IF on the immune system has been considered in some detail in a preceding section. Exactly how IF controls the growth of tumours *in vivo* is not clear, although modulation of the immune system is a strong possibility. Much work is still required to establish the precise mechanism whereby IF affects tumours, in order to optimise treatment conditions.

In summary, nonspecific immunotherapy has proved highly successful in animal models designed to prove its efficacy. Early clinical trials were promising but critical appraisal of these and subsequent studies reveals only marginal benefit. The attraction of nonspecific immunotherapy is that it avoids the necessity for preparation of a specific vaccine for each tumour or tumour type; it augments and potentiates the natural defences of the host. Nonspecific immunotherapy clearly merits further study.

9.2. Specific immunotherapy

A prerequisite for successful specific immunotherapy is the expression on tumour cells of a tumour-associated antigen against which a rejection response can be initiated. This may involve the induction of specific cytolytic T-lymphocytes or possibly antibody. With immunogenic animal tumours adjuvant therapy using BCG mixed with tumour cells enhances specific transplant resistance [117, 118]. Successful BCG-induced 'contact' therapy has been shown in many experimental tumour systems. Thus, viable tumour cells mixed with BCG and injected into appropriate recipients, stimulates non-specific defence mechanisms to suppress tumour growth. As a consequence, and providing the tumour expresses appropriate cell surface antigens, successful contact therapy can lead to the induction of specific systemic immunity and destruction of tumour cells at other body sites. With immunogenic rat hepatomas contact therapy given up to 6 days following inoculation of viable hepatoma cells alone results in successful therapy of the primary inoculum (Jones and Rees, unpublished observations), although it must be appreciated that such effects only occur under optimum experimental conditions. This approach to the treatment of human cancer requires that tumours possess a transplantation rejection antigen, and since at present this is not firmly established, the application of specific therapy of human cancer is limited.

In instances where human tumour antigens are expressed, treatments can be sought to enhance specific antitumour responses, in the hope of redressing the balance in favour of host survival. It has proved possible to generate clonal expansion of sensitised T-lymphocytes *in vitro* in medium containing a T-cell growth factor [119]. In addition, application of this technology to the *in vitro* generation of large numbers of lymphocytes possessing either specific or non-specific antitumour reactivity, may serve as an alternative to active stimulation of immune reactions in cancer patients.

The failure of direct administration of immunotherapeutic reagents may be due in part to intrinsic defects in the ability of the patient's immune system to respond. The employment of passive immunotherapy is an area of research which has met with success in experimental systems [120]; clearly much work is still needed in this area, especially using models more relevant to human cancer which metastasise naturally from the site of primary tumour implantation.

The use of tumour-specific antibody in the therapy of malignant disease has lost favour, due in the main to results in animal systems. However, the idea of using specific antitumour antibody to target other toxic reagents, such as drugs, to the site of tumour growth may still prove viable, and experimentally at least beneficial effects have been shown using this technique [121, 122, 123]. The application of this treatment in the therapy of human cancer may perhaps be more difficult, since in the past a reliable method of producing sufficient quantities of antibody with the desired specificity has not been available. Recently, many groups of workers have used hybridomas systems to generate large quantities of monoclonal antibody for therapy [124, 125]. This research is in its infancy, but further work in this field could determine its therapeutic potential for the treatment of the human disease.

10. Immune reactivity as a monitor of tumour response

In section 8 we considered the use of tests of tumour-specific immune reactivity in the diagnosis of cancer. In this section the use of such tests in the clinical monitoring of tumour growth will be summarised. At the outset it must be emphasised, however, that the problems of reproducibility and sensitivity alluded to in section 8 are further compounded by the surgical, radiotherapeutic, and chemotherapeutic procedures to which cancer patients are exposed during the clinical management of their disease. These procedures inevitably modulate the function of the immune system directly; any measured changes in tumour-specific immune reactivity may be due either to the patient's treatment or to the progression or resolution of their disease. This contrasts with the use of immunoassays for tumour marker substances (e.g. carcinoembryonic antigen, α-fetoprotein, chorionic gonadotrophin); the concentration of these substances in body fluids varies in accordance with the tumour burden and is largely independent of the effects of therapy on the patient's immune system.

In an assay of lymphocyte cytotoxicity in bladder cancer patients it was found that 44% of patients with proven recurrent tumour gave a false-negative result [131]; this is an unacceptably high incidence, rendering the test relatively useless for clinical purposes. Lymphocyte microcytotoxicity assays in an earlier study [132] had shown, however, that although lymphocytotoxicity required the presence of viable tumour or tumour-derived antigens, the presence of a large tumour or metastases was associated with a diminished effect.

In a study of lymphocyte transformation in response to specific and non-specific mitogens in melanoma patients, the use of BCG to promote immunocompetence did not lead to enhanced lymphocyte responsiveness even when it was initially diminished [133]; any change in lymphocyte reactivity appeared to be related to tumour burden.

Delayed hypersensitivity responses to skin testing with dinitrochlorobenzene (DNCB) are often depressed in patients with disseminated tumour (melanomas and soft tissue and skeletal sarcomas); persistence of this anergic state or conversion of a reactive to an anergic state is associated with a high incidence of recurrent tumours [134]. In breast cancer parameters of depressed cell-mediated immunity have been shown to be of little clinical value because significant depression only occurs in the terminal stages of the disease [135].

Of questionably greater promise in this regard is the leukocyte adherence inhibition (LAI) test (see section 8.4). LAI appears to diminish progressively with tumour burden in breast cancer [136] and some other malignancies. When several months have elapsed after mastectomy most patients have a negative LAI. A persistence or reappearance of LAI may be associated with an increased risk of recurrence. The diminished LAI seen terminally is probably due to 'blocking' by excess tumour antigen.

In summary, perturbations in specific and nonspecific immune reactivity during tumour growth may be due to either the undesirable immunosuppressive effects of surgery, radiotherapy and chemotherapy or to genuine fluctuations in tumour burden. More work is necessary to further refine and evaluate these techniques. At the present time, however, clinical applications are confined to those institutions where research groups have built up considerable expertise in the conduct and interpretation of these somewhat fickle tests.

References

1. Everson TC, Cole WH: Spontaneous regression of cancer. Philadelphia: Saunders, 1966.
2. Woglom WH: Immunity to transplantable tumours. Cancer Rev 4:129–214, 1929.
3. Gross L: Intradermal immunization of C3H mice against a sarcoma that originated in an animal of the same line. Cancer Res 13:835–837, 1943.
4. Foley EJ: Antigenic properties of methylcholanthrene-induced tumours in mice of the strain of origin. Cancer Res 13:835–837, 1953.
5. Prehn RT, Main JM: Immunity to methylcholanthrene-induced sarcomas. J Natl Cancer Inst 18:768–778, 1957.
6. Rees RC, Potter CW: *In vivo* studies of cell-mediated and humoral immune response to adenovirus 12-induced tumour cells. Arch Ges Virusforsch 41:116–126, 1973.
7. Price MR, Baldwin RW: Preparation of aminoazo dye induced rat hepatoma membrane fractions retaining tumour specific antigen. Br J Cancer 30:382–393, 1974.
8. Price MR, Baldwin RW: Immunogenic properties of rat hepatoma subcellular fractions. Br J Cancer 30:394–400, 1974.
9. Hellstrom I, Hellstrom KE, Pierce GE, Yang JPS: Cellular and humoral immunity to different types of human neoplasms. Nature 220:1352–1354, 1968.
10. Takasugi M, Mickey MR, Terasaki PI: Reactivity of lymphocytes from normal persons on cultured tumour cells. Cancer Res 33:2898–2902, 1973.
11. Herberman RB, Holden HT: Natural cell-mediated immunity. Adv Cancer Res 27:-305–377, 1978.
12. Underwood JCE: Lymphoreticular infiltration in human tumours: prognostic and biological implications: A review. Br J Cancer 30:538–548, 1974.
13. Underwood JCE, Carr I: The ultrastructure of lymphoreticular cells in non-lymphoid human neoplasms. Virchows Arch Abt B Zellpath 12:39–50, 1972.
14. Nind APP, Nairn RC, Rolland JM, Guli EPG, Hughs ESR: Lymphocyte anergy in patients with carcinoma. Br J Cancer 28:108–117, 1973.
15. Archibald RB, Frenster JH: Quantitative ultrastructural analysis of in vivo lymphocyte Reed-Sternberg cell interactions in Hodgkin's disease. Natl Cancer Inst Monogr 36:239–245, 1973.
16. Leffell MS, Coggin JH: Common transplantation antigens on methylcholanthrene-induced murine sarcomas detected by three assays of tumour rejection. Cancer Res 37:4112–4119, 1977.
17. Economou GC, Takeichi N, Boone CW: Common tumour rejection antigens in methylcholanthrene-induced squamous cell carcinomas of mice detected by tumour protection and a radioisotopic footpad assay. Cancer Res 37:37–41, 1977.

18. Kadhim SA, Rees RC: T-lymphocyte mediated tumor rejection of a C51Bl mouse sarcoma: Characterization of effector cells by *in vivo* adoptive transfer assay. Submitted for publication.
19. Rees RC, Price MR, Baldwin RW: Oncodevelopmental antigen expression in chemical carcinogenesis. Methods Cancer Res 18:99–133, 1979.
20. Coggin JH, Ambrose KR: Embryonic and fetal determinants on virally and chemically induced tumors. Methods Cancer Res 18:371–389, 1979.
21. Hewitt HB, Blake ER, Walder AS: A critique of the evidence for active host defence against cancer based on personal studies of 27 murine tumours of spontaneous origin. Br J Cancer 33:241–259, 1976.
22. Wrathmell AB, Alexander P: Immunogenicity of a rat leukaemia of spontaneous origin (SAL). Br J Cancer 33:181–186, 1976.
23. Vasa-Thomas KA, Ambrose KR, Bellomy BB, Coggin JH: Characterization of immune responses to spontaneous hamster lymphomas. J Natl Cancer Inst 58:1287–1293, 1977.
24. Hammond WG, Fisher JC, Rolley RT: Tumour-specific transplantation immunity to spontaneous mouse tumors. Surgery 62:124–133, 1967.
25. Hewitt HB: The choice of animal tumours for experimental studies of cancer therapy. Adv Cancer Res 27:149–200, 1978.
26. Hewitt HB: A critical examination of the foundations of immunotherapy for cancer. Clin Radiol 30:361–369, 1979.
27. Law LW, Rogers MJ, Appella E: Tumor antigens on neoplasms induced by chemical carcinogens and by DNA- and RNA-containing viruses: properties of the solubilized antigens. Adv Cancer Res 32:201–235, 1980.
28. Natori T, Law LW, Appella E: Biologic and biochemical properties of detergent-solubilized tumor-specific transplantation antigen from a simian virus 40-induced neoplasm: Brief communication. J Natl Cancer Inst 59:1331–1333, 1977.
29. Pellis NR, Kahan BD: Specific tumor immunity induced with soluble materials: restricted range of antigen dose and of challenge tumor load for immunoprotection. J Immunol 115:1717–1722, 1975.
30. Pasternak L, Pasternak G, Karsten U: Immunogenicity of soluble extracts from a UV light-induced mouse sarcoma. Cancer Immunol Immunother 3:273–275, 1978.
31. Bubenich J, Indrova N, Nemeckova S, Malkovsky M, Von Broen B, Palek V, Anderlikov T: Solublised tumour associated antigens of methylcholanthrene-induced mouse sarcomas. Comparative studies by *in vitro* sensitisation of lymph node cells, macrophage electrophoretic mobility assay and transplantation tests. Int J Cancer 21:348-355, 1978.
32. Price MR, Preston VE, Robins RA, Zoller M, Baldwin RW: Induction of immunity to chemically-induced rat tumours by cellular or soluble antigens. Cancer Immunol Immunother 3:247–252, 1978.
33. Kurth R, Fenyer EM, Klein E, Essex M: Cell-surface antigens induced by RNA tumour viruses. Nature 279:197–201, 1979.
34. Hellstrom I: A Colony inhibition (CI) technique for demonstration of tumour cell destruction by lymphoid cells *in vitro*. Int J Cancer 2:65–68, 1967.
35. Takasugi M, Klein E: A microassay for cell-mediated immunity. Transplantation 9:219–227, 1970.
36. Brookes CG, Rees RC, Baldwin RW: Studies on the microtoxicity test. I. Evidence that the effects of normal lymphocytes on tumour cell growth in microtest plates are caused by non-immunological modifications of the culture media. Int J Cancer 18:778–786, 1976.
37. Powell AE, Sloss AM, Smith RN, Makley JT, Hubay CA: Specific responsiveness of leukocytes to soluble extracts of human tumours. Int J Cancer:905–913, 1975.
38. Sinkovics JG, Campos LT, Kay HD, Cabines JR, Gonzalez F, Loh KK, Ervin F, Gyorkey F: Immunological studies with human sarcomas. Effects of immunisation and chemo-

therapy on cell- and antibody-mediated immune reactions. In: Immunological aspects of neoplasia. Baltimore: Williams and Wilkins Co., 1975, pp 367–401.

39. Mavligit GM, Gutterman JU, McBride GM, Hersh EM: Cell-mediated immunity to human solid tumours *in vitro* detection by lymphocyte blastogenic responses to cell-associated and solubilised tumour antigens. Natl Cancer Inst Monogr 37:167, 1973.
40. Cohen AM, Ketcham AS, Morton DL: Tumour-specific cellular cytotoxicity of human sarcomas. Evidence for a cell-mediated immune response to a common sarcoma cell-surface antigen. J Natl Cancer Inst 50:585–589, 1973.
41. Gainor BJ, Forbes JT, Enneking WF, Smith RT: Specific antigen stimulated lymphocytes proliferation in osteosarcoma. Cancer 37: 743–750, 1976.
42. Rella W, Kotz R, Arbes H, Leber H: Tumour-specific immunity in sarcoma patients. Oncology 34:219–223, 1977.
43. Vanky F, Argov S: Human tumour - lymphocyte interaction *in vitro*. VII. Blastogenesis and generation of cytotoxicity against autologous tumour biopsy cells are inhibited by interferon. Int J Cancer 26:405–411, 1980.
44. Vanky F, Stjernsward J: Lymphocyte stimulation. In: Immunodiagnosis of cancer, Herberman RB, McIntire KR (eds). New York: Marcel Dekker Inc., 1979, pp 889–1032.
45. Vose BM, Vanky F, Fopp M, Klein E: *In vitro* generation of cytotoxicity against autologous human tumour biopsy cells. Int J Cancer 21:588–593, 1978.
46. Wells SA Jr, Burdich JF, Christiansen C, Ketcham AS, Atkins P: Demonstration of tumour associated delayed cutaneous hypersensitivity reactions in patients with lung cancer and in patients with carcinoma of the cervix. Natl Cancer Inst Mong 37:197–203, 1973.
47. Hollinshead AC, Stewart THM, Herberman RB: Delayed-hypersensitivity reactions to soluble membrane antigens of human malignant lung cells. J Natl Cancer Inst 52:327–338, 1974.
48. Bell CE: Human lung cancer plasma membrane antigens. In: Serological analysis of human cancer antigens, Rosenberg SA (ed). New York: Academic Press, 1980, pp 239–251.
49. Shiku H, Takahashi T, Carey T, Resnick L, Pfreundschah M, Ueda R, Oettgen HF, Old LJ: Definition of cell surface antigens of human malignant melanoma, astrocytoma, and renal cancer by typing with autologous serum. In: Serologic analysis of human cancer antigens, Rosenberg SA (ed). New York: Academic Press, 1980, pp 305–337.
50. Hawrylko E, Mackaness GB: Immunopotentiation with BCG IV. Factors affecting the magnitude of an anti-tumour response. J Natl Cancer Inst 51:1683–1688, 1973.
51. Fogel M, Gorelick E, Segal S, Cohen IR, Feldman M: Demonstration of antigenic differences between a local tumour of Lewis lung carcinoma (3LL) and its pulmonary metastases. Isr J Med Sci 13:1032, 1977.
52. Bosslet K, Schirrmacher V, Shantz G: Tumour metastases and cell-mediated immunity in a model system in DBA/2 mice. VI. Similar specificity patterns of protective anti-tumour immunity *in vivo* and of cytolytic T cells *in vitro*. Int J Cancer 24:303–313, 1979.
53. Frost P, Kerbel RS: Immunoselection *in vitro* of a non-metastatic variant from a highly metastatic tumour. Int J Cancer 27:381–385, 1981.
54. Chow DA, Greenberg AH: The generation of tumour heterogeneity *in vivo*. Int J Cancer 25:261–265, 1980.
55. Schirrmacher V, Shantz G, Clauer K, Komitowski D, Zimmermann HP, Lohmann-Mathes M: Tumour metastases and cell mediated immunity in a model system in DBA/2 mice. I. Tumour invasiveness *in vitro* and metastases formation *in vivo*. Int J Cancer 23:233–244, 1979.
56. Gorelick E, Fogel M, Segal S, Feldman M: Tumour-associated antigenic differences between the primary and the descendant metastatic tumour cell populations. J Supramolec Struct 12:385–402, 1979.

57. Faldt R, Ankerst J: Tumour-associated humoral cytotoxicity in patients with acute myelogenous leukemia before and after chemotherapy. Int J Cancer 20:824–833, 1977.
58. Brunner KT, Mauel J, Cerottini JC, Chapuis B: Quantitative assay of the lytic action of immune lymphoid cells on ^{51}Cr-labelled allogeneic target cells *in vitro*; inhibition by isoantibody and by drugs. Immunology 14:181–196, 1978.
59. Rosenberg EB, Herberman RB, Levine PH, Halterman RH, McCoy JL, Wanderlick JR: Lymphocyte cytotoxicity reactions to leukemia-associated antigens in identical tumours. Int J Cancer 9:648–658, 1972.
60. Heppner G, Henry E, Stobbach L, Cummings F, McDonough E, Calabresi P: Problems in the clinical use of the microcytotoxicity assay for measuring cell-mediated immunity to tumour cells. Cancer Res 35:1931–1937, 1975.
61. Peter H, Pavie-Fischer J, Fridman W, Aubert C, Cesarini JP, Roubin R, Kourilsky FM: Cell-mediated cytoxicity *in vitro* of human lymphocytes against a tissue culture melanoma cell line (IGR_3). J Immunol 115:539–548, 1975.
62. Kiessling R, Klein E, Wigzell H: Natural killer cells in the mouse. I. Cytotoxic cells with specificity for mouse leukemia cells. Specificity and distribution according to genotype. Eur J Immunol 5:112–117, 1975.
63. Herberman RB, Djeu JY, Kay HD, Ortaldo JR, Riccardi C, Bonnard GD, Holden HT, Fagnani R, Santoni A, Puccetti P: Natural killer cells: characteristics and regulation of activity. Immunol Rev 44:43–70, 1979.
64. Herberman RB, Nunn ME, Holden HT, Lavrin DH: Natural cytotoxic reactivity of mouse lymphoid cells against syngeneic and allogeneic tumours. II. Characterization of effector cells. Int J Cancer 16:230–239, 1975.
65. Santoli D, Koprowski H: Mechanism of activation of human natural killer cells against tumour and virus-infected cells. Immunol Rev 44:125–163, 1979.
66. Riccardi C, Santoni A, Barlozzari T, Herberman RB: *In vivo* natural reactivity of mice against tumor cells. Int J Cancer 25:475–486, 1980.
67. Rees RC, Reynolds C, Herberman RB: Natural cytotoxicity of rat lymphoid cells towards solid tumour targets grown *in vitro*. In preparation.
68. West WH, Cannon GB, Kay HD, Bonnard GD, Herberman RB: Natural cytotoxic reactivity of human lymphocytes against a myeloid cell line: characterization of effector cells. J Immunol 118:355–361, 1977.
69. Einhorn S, Blomgren H, Strander H: Interferon and spontaneous cytotoxicity in man. V. Enhancement of spontaneous cytotoxicity in patients receiving human leukocyte interferon. Int J Cancer 26:419–428, 1980.
70. Djeu JY, Heinbaugh JA, Holden HT, Herberman RB: Augmentation of mouse natural killer cell activity by interferon and interferon inducers. J Immunol 122:175–181, 1979.
71. Gidlund M, Orn A, Wigzell H, Senik A, Gresser I: Enhanced NK cell activity in mice injected with interferon and interferon inducers. Nature 273:759–761, 1978.
72. Herberman RB, Nunn ME, Holden HT, Staal S, Djeu JY: Augmentation of natural cytotoxic reactivity of mouse lymphoid cells against syngeneic and allogenic target cells. Int J Cancer 19:555–564, 1977.
73. Trinchieri G, Santoli D: Anti-viral activity induced by culturing lymphocytes with tumor-derived of virus-transformed cells. J Exp Med 147:1314–1333, 1978.
74. Einhorn S, Bromgren H, Strander H: Interferon and spontaneous cytotoxicity in man. I. Enhancement of the spontaneous cytotoxicity of peripheral lymphocytes by human leukocyte interferon. Int J Cancer 22:405–412, 1978.
75. Herberman RB: Augmentation of NK activity. In: Natural cell-mediated immunity against tumors, Herberman RB (ed). New York: Academic Press, 1980, pp 239–251.
76. Burnet FM: The concept of immunological surveillance. Prog Exp Tumour Res 13:1–27, 1970.

77. Rygaard J, Povlsen CO: The nude mouse vs the hypothesis of immunological surveillance. Transplant Rev 28:43–61, 1976.
78. Riesenfeld I, Tufveson G, Alm GV: Lymphoma development from transplanted murine leukaemia virus infected organ cultured thymuses: Inhibitory effect of *in vitro* interferon treatment. Int J Cancer 25:529–534, 1980.
79. Haller O, Hansson M, Kiessling R, Wigzell H: Role of non-conventional natural killer cells in resistance against syngeneic tumour cells *in vivo*. Nature 270:609–611, 1977.
80. Harman RC, Clarke EA, O'Toole C, Wickler LS: Resistance of H2-heterozygous mice to parental tumours. I. Hybrid resistance and natural cytotoxicity to EL-4 are controlled by the H-2D Hh-1 region. Immunogenetics 41:601–607, 1977.
81. Herberman RB, Nunn ME, Lavrin DH: Natural cytotoxic reactivity of mouse lymphoid cells against syngeneic and allogeneic tumours. I. Distribution or reactivity and specificity. Int J Cancer 16:216–229, 1975.
82. Becker S, Klein E: Decreased 'natural killer' – NK – effect in tumour-bearing mice and its relation to the immunity against oncornavirus determined cell surface antigens. Eur J Immunol 6:892–898, 1976.
83. Gerson JM, Holden HT, Bonnard GD, Herberman RB: Natural killer cell (NK) activity in murine and human tumors. Proc Amer Assoc Cancer Res 20:238, 1979.
84. Pross HF, Baines MG: Spontaneous human lymphocyte-mediated cytoxicity against tumour target cells. I. The effect of malignant disease. Int J Cancer 18:593–604, 1976.
85. Takasugi M, Ramseyer A, Takasugi J: Decline of natural nonselective cell-mediated cytotoxicity in patients with tumor progression. Cancer Res 37:413–418, 1977.
86. Hawrylowicz CM, Rees RC, Hancock BW, Potter CW: Depressed natural killer cell activity in patients with malignant lymphoma and failure of NK cells to respond to interferon treatment *in vitro*. Eur J Cancer 1982 (in press).
87. Britten V, Rees RC, Clegg A, Smith GT, Potter CW, Fox M, Williams JL: Natural killer cell activity and response to phytohaemagglutinin compared with the histological diagnosis of patients with transitional cell carcinoma of the bladder. Br J Urol 1982 (in press).
88. Vose BM, Moore M: Suppressor cell activity of lymphocytes infiltrating human lung and breast tumours. Int J Cancer 24:579–585, 1977.
89. Vose BM: Natural killers in human cancer: activity of tumor-infiltrating and draining node lymphocytes. In: Natural cell-mediated immunity against tumors, Herberman RB (ed). New York: Academic Press, 1980, pp 1081–1097.
90. Gerson JM: Systemic and in situ natural killer activity in tumor-bearing mice and patients with cancer. In: Natural cell-mediated immunity against tumors, Herberman RB (ed). New York: Academic Press, 1980, pp 1047–1062.
91. Perussia B, Trinchieri G: Inactivation of natural killer cell cytotoxic activity after interaction with target cells. J Immunol 126:754–758, 1981.
92. Stutman O, Figarella EF, Paige CJ, Lattime EC: Natural cytotoxic (NC) cells against solid tumors in mice: general characteristics and comparison to natural killer (NK) cells. In: Natural cell-mediated immunity against tumors, Herberman RB (ed). Academic Press, 1980, pp 187–229.
93. Stutman O, Paige CJ, Figarella EF: Natural cytotoxic cells against solid tumours in mice. I. Strain and age distribution and target cell susceptibility. J Immunol 121:1819–1826, 1978.
94. Paige CJ, Figarella EF, Cuttino MJ, Cahan A, Stutman O: Natural cytoxic cells against solid tumours in mice. II. Some characteristics of the effector cells. J Immunol 121:1827–1835, 1978.
95. Keller R: Regulatory capacities of mononuclear phagocytes with particular reference to natural immunity against tumors. In: Natural cell-mediated immunity against tumors. Herberman RB (ed). New York: Academic Press, 1980, pp 1219–1269.

96. Mantovani A, Peri G, Polentarutti N, Allavena P: Natural cytotoxicity on tumor cells of human monocytes and macrophages. In: Natural cell-mediated immunity against tumors, Herberman RB (ed). New York: Academic Press, 1980, pp 1271–1293.
97. Currie GA, Basham C: Activated macrophages release a factor which lyses malignant cells but not normal cells. J Exp Med 142:1600–1605, 1975.
98. Aksamit RR, Kim KJ: Macrophage cell lines produce a cytotoxin. J Immunol 122:1785–1790, 1979.
99. Noar D: Suppressor cells: permitters and promoters of malignancy? Adv Cancer Res 29:45–125, 1979.
100. Penn I: Tumours arising in organ transplant recipients. Adv Cancer Res 28:31–61, 1978.
101. Kamo I, Friedman H: Immunosuppression and the role of suppressive factors in cancer. Adv Cancer Res 25:271–321, 1977.
102. Badger AM, Cooperband SR, Merluzzi VJ: Suppressive immuno activity of ascitic fluid from patients with cancer metastatic to the peritoneum. Cancer Res 37:1220–1226, 1977.
103. Herberman RB: Immunologic approaches to the diagnosis of cancer. Cancer 37:548–862, 1976.
104. Herberman RB: Delayed hypersensitivity skin reactions to antigens on human tumours. Cancer 34:1469–1473, 1974.
105. Forrester JA, Dando PM, Smith WJ, Turberville C: Failure to confirm the macrophage electrophoretic mobility test in cancer. Br J Cancer 36:537–544, 1977.
106. Caspary EA, Field EJ: Specific lymphocyte sensitisation in cancer: is there a common antigen in human malignant neoplasia? Br Med J ii:613–617, 1971.
107. Halliday WS, Maluish AE, Isbister WH: Detection of anti-tumour cell-mediated immunity and serum blocking factors in cancer patients by the leucocyte adherance inhibition test. Br J Cancer 29:31–35, 1974.
108. Goodnight JE, Morton DL: Immunotherapy of cancer: current status. Prog Exp Tumour Res 25:61–88, 1980.
109. Currie GA, Basham C: Serum mediated inhibition of the immunological reactions of the patient to his own tumour: a possible role for circulating antigen. Br J Cancer 26:427–438, 1972.
110. Ruckdeschel JC, Codish SD, Stranahan A, McKneally MF: Postoperative empyema improves survival in lung cancer: documentation and analysis of a natural experiment. N Engl J Med 287:1013–1017, 1972.
111. Mathé G, Amiel JL, Schwarzenberg L, Schneider M, Cattan A, Schlumberger JR, Hayat M, Vassal F: Active immunotherapy for acute lymphoblastic leukaemia. Lancet i:697–699, 1969.
112. McKneally MF, Maver CM, Kausel HW: Intrapleural BCG stimulation in lung cancer. Lancet i:593, 1977.
113. Morton DL, Eilber FR, Holmes EC, Hunt JS, Ketcham AS, Silverstein MJ, Sparks FC: BCG immunotherapy of malignant melanoma: survey of a seven-year experience. Ann Surg 180:635–643, 1974.
114. Sparks FC, Silverstein MJ, Hunt JS, Haskell CM, Pilch YH, Morton DL: Complications of BCG immunotherapy in patients with cancer. N Engl J Med 289:827–830, 1973.
115. Spitler LE: BCG, levamisole and transfer factor in the treatment of cancer. Prog Exp Tumour Res 25:178–192, 1980.
116. Rojas AF, Mickiewicz E, Feierstein JN, Glait H, Olivari AJ: Levamisole in advanced human breast cancer. Lancet i:211–213, 1976.
117. Mausawy KM, Rees RC, Potter CW: Immunogenic properties of hamster tumours of herpesvirus hominis aetiology. Cancer Immunol Immunother 8:119–126, 1980.

118. Baldwin RW, Pimm MV: BCG in tumor immunotherapy. Adv Cancer Res 28:91–147, 1978.
119. Cheever MA, Greenberg PD, Fefer A: Specific adoptive therapy of established leukemia with syngeneic lymphocytes sequentially immunized *in vivo* and *in vitro* and non-specifically expanded by culture with interleukin 2. J Immunol 126:1318–1322, 1981.
120. Rosenberg SA, Terry WD: Passive immunotherapy of cancer in animals and man. Adv Cancer Res 25:323–388, 1977.
121. Ghose T, Norvell ST, Guclu A, Cameron D, Bodurtha A, MacDonald AS: Immunochemotherapy of cancer with chlorambucil-carrying antibody. Br Med J 3:495–499, 1972.
122. Ghose T, Nigam SP: Antibody as carrier of chlorambucil. Cancer 29:1398–1400, 1972.
123. Flechner I: The cure and concomitant immunization of mice bearing Ehrlich ascites tumors by treatment with an antibody-alkylating agent complex. Eur J Cancer 9:741–745, 1973.
124. Nadler LM, Stashenko P, Hardy R, Kaplan WD, Button LN, Kufe DW, Autman KH, Schlossman SF: Serotherapy of a patient with a monoclonal antibody directed against a human lymphoma-associated antigen. Cancer Res 40:3147–3154, 1980.
125. Deng C, Terasaki PI, El-Awar N, Billing R, Cicciarelli J, Lagasse L: Cytotoxic monoclonal antibody to a human leiomyosarcoma. Lancet i:403–405, 1981.
126. Old LJ, Stockert E: Immunogenetics of cell surface antigens of mouse leukemia. Ann Rev Genet II:127–160, 1977.
127. Kurth R, Bauer H: Cell-surface antigens induced by avian RNA tumor viruses: detection by a cytotoxic microassay. Virology 47:426–433, 1972.
128. Essex M, Klein G, Snyder SP, Harrold JB: Correlation between humoral antibody and regression of tumours induced by feline sarcoma virus. Nature 233:195–196, 1971.
129. Ting CC, Shiu G, Rodrigues D, Herberman RB: Cell-mediated immunity to friend virus-induced leukemia. Cancer Res 34:1684–1687, 1974.
130. Kunkel LA, Welsh RM: Metabolic inhibitors render 'resistant' target cells sensitive to natural killer cell mediated lysis. Int J Cancer 27:73–80, 1981.
131. Vilien M, Wolf H, Rasmussen F: Follow-up investigations of bladder cancer patients by titration of natural and specific lymphocyte-mediated cytotoxicity; prognostic significance of specific reactivity. Cancer Immunol Immunother 10:171–180, 1981.
132. O'Toole CO, Perlmann P, Unsgaard B, Moberger G, Edsmyr F: Cellular immunity to human urinary bladder carcinoma. I. Correlation to clinical stage and radiotherapy. Int J Cancer 10:77–91, 1977.
133. Golub SH, Forsythe AB, Morton DL: Sequential examination of lymphocyte proliferative capacity in patients with malignant melanoma receiving BCG immunotherapy. Int J Cancer 19:18–26, 1977.
134. Eilber FR, Nizza JA, Morton DL: Sequential evaluation of general immune competence in cancer patients: correlation with clinical course. Cancer 35:660–665, 1975.
135. Nemoto T, Han T, Minowada J. Angkur V, Chamberlain A, Dao TL: Cell-mediated immune status of breast cancer patients: evaluation by skin tests, lymphocyte stimulation and counts of rosette-forming cells. J Natl Cancer Inst 53:641–645, 1974.
136. Flores M, Marti JH, Grosser N, MacFarlane JK, Thompson DMP: An overview: antitumour immunity in breast cancer assayed by tube leukocyte adherence inhibition. Cancer 39:484–505, 1977.

SUBJECT INDEX

Printed in the United States
900200004B

9 789024 727124